# Perfect Bones

A Six-Point Plan
to Promote
Healthy Bones

Pamela Levin, R.N.

Technical Editing by Corey Cameron Cooper, D.C., C.C.S.P.
Proofreading by Rita Samols
Cover design and illustration by Lightbourne, Copyright 1999
Book Design and Composition by Classic Typography

Library of Congress Catalog Card Number: 99-96171

    Levin, Pamela, R.N.
    Perfect bones, a six-point plan to promote healthy bones / by Pamela Levin
    p. cm.
    Includes bibliographical references and index
    ISBN 0-9672718-0-0

1. Osteoporosis—Popular Works 2. Health 3. Nutrition 4. Alternative Medicine 5. Medical Care—Philosophy 6. Clinical Nutrition 7. Holistic Medicine 8. Women—Health 9. Title

Printed in the United States of America
The Nourishing Company/ Post Office Box 1429/ Ukiah, California 95482

In gratitude to the One Who nourishes all.

✒ Contents

Part Three

~ Foreword

Pam's genius in the professional community is no longer the secret of a few. She possesses a framework of intelligence supported by the necessary knowledge and experience of a highly skilled student of clinical nutrition and C.R.A.™ technology.

Her book and writings indicate she has understood what true health care really is—taking care of the whole person as a living physical organism.

Pam is committed. She accepts no excuses, only results. She is eager to lead the way with great anticipation, thus creating incredible opportunities for professional success. She believes there are no hopeless situations, only those who think hopelessly.

Pam's achievement in this book is based not only on her knowledge of clinical nutrition and C.R.A.™, but also on her contributions to the field of human development and emotional health. It is obvious her talents will give new life to the alternative health community.

She believes only a powerful commitment can break one out of self-defeating patterns. May her compelling motto, Vis Medicatrix Natural—The Healing Power of Nature—be the challenge for those who wish to outlive their dreams.

DICK VERSENDAAL, D.C.

∽ Preface

Everybody wants perfect bones, yet fewer and fewer of us have them, especially as we age. Estimates say that in the next few years, 45 million of us will be at risk for developing osteoporosis, a number expected to triple over the next 60 years (to 135 million), and that more of us will die from osteoporosis-related problems than from the top two killers (heart disease and breast cancer) put together!

But it's not only adults—even the next generation is affected. Experts are currently lobbying the World Health Organization to have osteoporosis declared a pediatric onset disease! Is there anything to be done? Is good bone health simply luck, or fate, or some secret known only to a select few? Must we simply resign ourselves to this awful, debilitating, and ultimately death-producing state?

The premise of this book is that indeed, there is much we can do, that the power to have healthy bones is in our own hands, and that the choices we make on a daily basis are central to the outcome for our bones. How is this so?

Osteoporosis has long been considered a disease, the inference being that it results from a body that simply malfunctions, as if such a breakdown were an event about which there is nothing to be done. But if we view osteoporosis as a *solution* to a bodily problem, a demonstration of the body's natural healing ability, that hopelessness can change. Sick bones are the body's answer to how to maintain homeostatic balance in the face of increasingly difficult challenges. When our bodies rob our bones of their life-giving minerals, for example, they do so to provide these essential substances to areas such as our heart and circulatory system, that are more important for sustaining life. This infers that the key to maintaining healthy bones is to provide what the body needs for homeostatic balance so it doesn't have to rob bones to sustain life.

How can we know, then, that our bodies are out of balance and therefore robbing our bones? Finding out may seem a difficult task, for declining bone health has long been labeled the "silent disease." Yet, after completing only a little research, I uncovered 84 different clues that the body is robbing our bones to keep us alive! (See Chapter 1.)

Perhaps we need to rename this "silent disease" the "deaf ear" disease, and conclude that we need to learn, or rather relearn, how to listen.

The National Osteoporosis Foundation has put forth that the number one task before us to stem this tidal wave of sick-boned population is to prevent osteoporosis in the first place, and that the number one way to do this is through diet. Indeed, our nutritional states are the very bones of bone health.

It has been my great pleasure to take up the mantle of nutritional journalist, and gather within these pages the essence of how to go about achieving and maintaining this health-conferring state of nutritional balance. The point is to provide the body with a better way to maintain homeostatic balance than creating porous bones.

We have every reason to believe that the power is in our own hands to create osteoperfecta: Perfect Bones.

PAMELA LEVIN
Ukiah, California, 1999

∽ Acknowledgments

M y deep gratitude to those dedicated giants of clinical nutrition whose knowledge is gathered in these pages. From an earlier era, both Royal Lee, D.D.S., and Price Pottenger, D.D.S., stand out. From today, special thanks to both genius and generosity of:

Dick Versendaal, D.C., who created a systematized, simple and highly effective way to tap into the power of nature to heal;

Michael Dobbins, D.C., whose knowledge of nutritional functions and pathways is unparalleled;

Kim Sperry, C.N.C., who developed the vegetarian protocols listed in these pages, who patiently shared her considerable knowledge and who personally taught me C.R.A.™;

Mary Jane Mack, R.N., who took me under her protective wing, professionally, and mentored me, and whose friendly knowledge, support and expertise were a constant source of inspiration;

Dan Newell, N.C., for his presence, availability, specialized knowledge and willingness to consult;

Bruce West, D.C., for sharing his extensive knowledge and experience with so many, and with me in particular;

Lee Vagt, D.C., for his clinical expertise and for helping me begin my own healing path.

I also owe a special debt of gratitude to: Hogie Wycoff and Nancy Ellis, for nurturing the writer in me; Richard Lind, Atlanta Georgia, for his wise counsel and unending faith; Linda Simone, who so generously gave of her skills and herself; Ray Worster, for his early enthusiasm, faith and problem-solving support; Lynda Myers, for extending a friendly editorial pen to the initial draft; Stacey Johnson, for her faith and dedication; Rick Moon, for his reassurance and problem-solving proficiencies; Jack Howell, for his guidance and enthusiasm; and Laura Samartino, for her loving guidance and profound wisdom, which have been and continue to remain crucial to my well-being.

Thanks, too, to those who gave other forms of assistance when needed, each in a distinctive and decisive way: Jon Buis, Penny Neal, Barbara Minogue, Renee Rutledge, Carol Gieg, Oni LaGioia, Jennie Burnstad, Marie McGarity, Karen Warren, Gail Shahbaghlian, Joan, John and Enid Griswold and Renee Freeman.

Last, a special debt of gratitude to Corey Cameron Cooper, D.C., C.C.S.P., for expert and timely technical and text editing.

Part One

CHAPTER ONE

What Is Osteoporosis and Can It Be Reversed?

T he pain seared through my back like a bullet ripping through my spine, and it knocked me to the ground as fast. One moment I had been reaching for my handbag to board the last leg of a flight home; the next, I was on the floor of the airport lounge, consumed by painful back spasms so severe I was not only unable to get up, I was going into shock. But I had not been shot. Rather, my back muscles had suddenly seized up, pulling my spinal bones out of alignment when I reached for my bag.

How could this have come about? Resting safely in bed at home two days later, with the help of friends living near the airport and their chiropractor, I had plenty of time to review. I had noticed a certain tension during sleep. I'd dismissed this as relating to work conflicts. Then there were backaches. I'd assumed they were from lifting kids and gardening. Still, morning stiffness had progressed so that it took considerable time to get out of bed. I had become used to ignoring it and would quickly remind myself I wasn't as young as I used to be and try to forget it. I decided I needed to get in shape. Preparing for a run one day, I leaned over to tie my shoes and my back had seized up. I was unable to get out of bed for a week.

Other warning signs had been more insistent. Once, for example, I shattered a tooth while eating bean dip! I asked my dentist if this might relate to calcium deficiency and received a negative answer. When the second tooth shattered, I received the same

3

reply. One night after a 14-hour plane trip, I had stretched in bed and ruptured a disc in my lower back. During my recovery, I made all kinds of promises to myself that if I ever got better I'd be a really good girl and exercise no matter what. Meanwhile I felt hopeless, like I was doing something wrong and didn't know what.

Well-meaning family and friends began assorted campaigns. "You have to exercise every day!" insisted one. But by now even walking could make my back seize up. A friend concluded emphatically, "It's all in your mind." I only felt more hopeless. I balked when a concerned relative insisted I get a consultation with an orthopedic surgeon. I'd seen what had happened to my own mother: five major back surgeries beginning in her mid-forties and over 30 years of unrelenting pain the surgeries did not relieve. Failing to heal from the last surgical invasion, she continued to deteriorate until she finally died.

To placate my family, I agreed to an x-ray. After spending two weeks recovering from a bulging disc, I presented myself at the x-ray department. The technician instructed me to lie in the very position I already knew was foolhardy for my back. I objected, he insisted. I protested, he grew testy. Finally, I complied, reinjured the disc and spent another two weeks recovering. The x-ray results were inconclusive. Considering I was nearing 50, I thought this sounded positive.

But I didn't feel very positive about my impaired lifestyle. For example, I'd learned not to try to do anything physical much before noon, especially leaning over to make the bed. As the afternoon progressed, my body seemed to improve slowly and I could increase my activity level if I were cautious with every move. But that meant drastically limiting things I loved to do, trying to cram them all into the tiny window of opportunity near nightfall. And I felt so frail, like a leaf in the wind that could easily be blown away. I had even become fearful of walking in a crowd, afraid someone would jostle me and I'd be injured. I was beginning to think I should give up trying to have the life I wanted and just learn to 'go gently into that dark night.' Had I been a different personality or different age, perhaps my experience would have been different.

It certainly was for Carol Gieg, now a woman, but whose problems began in childhood. Activity had been so much a part of her youthful life that if her body was giving her signals that she was going over the edge of toleration, she either didn't listen or denied them. What she did do was keep going. After all, she was a young girl, and activity was her life. Kids have accidents sometimes, they fall, they bump, they get hit. But five fractures in six years? That became impossible to ignore. She sought medical help and continued her beloved activity. Then, she broke her hip! Her age: twenty-two.

These two scenarios, Carol's and mine, are but two different versions of a story with the same title: Osteoporosis. This is what it's like to lose your bones. Whether you decrease your activity to avoid injury or keep active and hurt yourself, the result is ultimately the same. Slowly and silently your abilities as a human are removed from you. Molecule by invisible molecule, atom by atom you lose your membership in the vertebrate world. You are slowly reduced to the realm of those undulant creatures adrift in the tides, for whom mere osmotic changes are a threat to existence, who are all nerves, jellylike. You are no longer capable of strong resolve or stamina; you are incapable of self-defense other than that of the mythical Medusa: producing such a fearful stare that anyone who looks into your eyes will immediately be turned to stone.

The Bones of the Problem

Are such accounts unusual or rare? The numbers speak for themselves. In the United States alone, out of some forty-six million people over the age of 45, it is estimated that some *twenty-five million* are dealing with their own versions of this story. Some sources claim 80% of these are women, while an Associated Press story reports a ratio of 6 female cases for every 1 male sufferer. The Osteoporosis and Related Bone Diseases National Resource Center reports that some "2 million American men have osteoporosis and another 3 million men are at risk for developing the disease." They add that osteoporosis "affects nearly half of all people— women and men—over the age of 75."[1] Indeed, in the United States, over 1.3 million fractures are attributed to osteoporosis each year!

According to the National Resource Center, Osteoporosis and Related Bone Diseases, this debilitating disease afflicts more women than heart disease, stroke, diabetes, breast cancer or arthritis. Fully half of all women between the ages of forty-five and seventy-five show signs of some degree of osteoporosis.[2] Another reports that 35% of women over age 60 and 10% of all men have osteoporosis![3] A pharmaceutical ad states one out of every four women over 50 is affected by osteoporosis.[4] In fact, a woman's risk of hip fracture is equal to her *combined* risk of breast, uterine and ovarian cancer. Statisticians conclude that the incidence of osteoporosis is expected to increase *threefold* over the next 60 years due to increased life expectancy, and to cost the U.S. more than *$10 billion* annually!

Are these numbers inflated or unreasonable? Might they be simply a miscalculation of demographic statistics? Apparently not. Bruce West, D.C., who has a long-standing clinical nutrition practice, concurs. "Most patients have osteoporosis," he says.

In the United States, the people who currently show signs of osteoporosis are only part of the picture. Since half the bone mass a woman loses occurs in the first 3 to 6 years after menopause begins, we can expect the number of sufferers to double by the year 2000 as some 20 million baby boomers enter the menopausal years.[5] And, in the years after menopause, by age 65 or 70 women and men lose bone mass at the same rate, and so can develop osteoporosis at the same rate. Author Gail Sheehy estimated that, before the end of the century, the number of people in the target age group (45 to 54) will increase by one half![6] However, even that turns out to be a conservative estimate. Current demographic research indicates that between 1990 and 2010, the number of women aged 45–54, the key menopausal group, is expected to grow by 73%. That translates to 3,500 women per day entering menopause!

Another part of this statistical picture, in a case of reverse sexism, is that men's bone health is often overlooked, partly because osteoporosis has been considered to be largely a disease affecting women. A second factor is that men frequently ignore and fail to communicate to their doctors the aches and pains often associated with the beginning stages of osteoporosis, and when they do, may be ignored. Third, the incidence of prostate dysfunction and disease is rapidly increasing, with testosterone production often affected as well. Fourth, medical treatments often negatively affect testosterone levels. And for men, healthy testosterone levels are essential for healthy bones.

In the United Kingdom, The Royal College of Physicians reports that "the incidence of hip fractures rose 254 percent between 1954 and 1983 and was then still rising . . . Every ten minutes someone in the UK has a fracture."[7]

In Australia, in 1996, osteoporosis caused over 20,000 hip fractures and 24,000 forearm fractures. It is expected that more that half of all Australian women over 60 and one third of all men will be affected by this debilitating and death-producing problem.[8]

Worldwide, osteoporosis is estimated to affect 200 million women. If men are affected at the ratio of one man for every six women, then there are some 33 million men who are also losing their bones. A recent Gallup poll revealed that, over age 50, men's risk of suffering an osteoporosis-related fracture is greater than that of developing clinical prostate cancer, and that one-third of those men who have a hip fracture will die within a year. The poll concluded that 1.5 million men have osteoporosis now, and that 3.5 million more are at high risk. Clearly, this is not only a "women's disease."[9]

Even the next generations are being affected. The University of Colorado, for example, is seeing so many signs of the disease in children that they are recommending that the World Health Organization declare osteoporosis a pediatric onset disease.

What is going on?

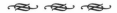

These two hundred million bodies have been undergoing a long, slow process known as demineralization, or loss of the mineral content which gives bones their strength, and that leads to porous bones. For many it began long before midlife. However, in midlife the results are sufficiently manifest to see the erosion that's been going on all the time.

While the word "demineralization" might sound innocuous enough, the diagnosis of osteoporosis can arouse bone-chilling dread. Simply put, osteoporosis means losing your bones. So what does this mean to me, you might wonder? In a word, everything.

Bones comprise 10% of your body. They are what hold the contents of your body into human form. Hidden deep within and essentially unseen, bones form the very essence of your human shape. Perhaps if bones were on the outside of your body like those of lobsters or crayfish, you would comprehend their relative state of health or disrepair much sooner.

But bones don't just provide a place for flesh and organs to attach, they are dynamic and alive. Their living tissue is composed of minerals, the levels of which fluctuate under the influence of other body functions.[10] Like branches of trees that provide a home for leaves and fruit and bring them the nourishment they need to grow and thrive, the bones of your skeleton provide a home for your flesh and organs and store nourishment for them.

A bone's living tissue is composed of three parts. The outside is hard, dense bone, analogous to tree bark, where calcium is stored in large amounts. The second layer is soft, spongy bone. The third layer is like the sap of the tree: it contains marrow, which manufactures the red blood cells that carry life-giving oxygen to every other cell in the body. Without that oxygen, all the metabolic fires of the rest of the body could not burn, and would smoulder and suffocate. Even a slight tamping of the bone marrow's manufacturing process can cause the lassitude and exhaustion we intuitively call "bone tired".

Bones have a detoxifying function in the body, too. Harmful elements such as lead, radium, fluorine and arsenic are removed from circulation and stored in bones and teeth.[11]

The red blood cells in the bone marrow are an integral part of the immune system. The marrow also manufactures antibodies, the white blood cells so small that a thimble can hold a quintillion! They also patrol the borders of the body to keep out or neutralize invaders. Bones also serve a health function crucial to the entire body: they are the storehouse for vital minerals needed to produce the enzymes on which every cell in the body depends.[12]

Strong bones are required for muscles to do their work. The ability to do anything, to act, to have strength, requires, first and foremost, healthy bones.

Because bones also record the history of the body, they are the focus of fields of study and research such as bioarcheology, forensic anthropology, human osteology, and environmental archeology. Bones are the last to remain of human remains, and whether they are well or poorly preserved, they chronicle stresses, physical hardships, and environmental pressures. According to the Museum of London Archaeology Service, long after you have left your bones behind, some future osteologist several thousand years from now will be able to "read" them and tell your age, race, gender, stature, individual pathology, and even reconstruct a demographic profile of your now-ancient population. They will be able to tell your family identity, ethnic or social group, and even interpret the nature of medicine you used and your level of hygiene. What we now know about ancient history—the era of the pyramids, or even the Stone Age—was gleaned from bones. Osteologists looking at the bones of former slaves, for example, have told us these bones are from people who worked so hard their muscles pulled off, along with a piece of bone, eventually killing some of them. So completely do bones reflect human existence that stories of ancient life can be reconstructed through excavated bones.

Bones tell the truth, even when it's different from what we want to believe. One truth they are telling is that the bones of people of all ages buried 300 years ago in England were in far better condition than those from skeletons of today. Bones have also revealed that osteoporosis was relatively uncommon until after World War I. The bones of people in "developing" countries reveal that they have far healthier bones than our own, despite the fact that these individuals consume less calcium per day than the average American.

Obviously, then, having sick bones is not an inevitable part of the human condition.[13] Some experts report that the increase in osteoporosis is due to the fact that people live longer. That's a disempowering idea that leaves only two unacceptable options: die early or degenerate slowly. Luckily, there's a lot of evidence that suggests the increase in osteoporosis is due to poor diet, bad food supply, increase in hysterectomies and orchiectomies, birth control pills, etc. And, there are many empowering actions to take to promote the possibility of both living long and staying healthy. The first of these is to listen to bodily signals.

How to Listen for the Silent Thief

So what is the truth your bones are telling you right now? What are the first indicators that you are on this downward evolutionary spiral? Are they sending a message that the creeping exhaustion, that vague ache, means a silent thief is at work deep inside you, stealing away your very bones? How do you detect the presence of such an invisible process now, while you can still do something about it? For most people who have begun this downward spiral, a kind of physical mousiness is a first indicator that the fate of the jellyfish might loom in their future. If that seems like little to go on, you're right. Osteoporosis is not called the "silent disease" because its onset is obvious. That means you'll need to infer its presence through the "at risk factors" listed below, which are compiled from a variety of sources.[14]

Warning Signs:

1. Feel depressed[15]
2. Regularly consume amounts of white flour and/or sugar
3. Consume soft drinks
4. Soft teeth
5. Habitually overeat
6. Tight jaw, clenched teeth and/or teeth grinding
7. Receding gums
8. Periodontal disease
9. Teeth loosening in sockets of jawbone
10. Jaw bone eroding
11. Shifting dental plates (indicating further jawbone erosion)
12. Tooth shattering
13. Plaque on the teeth
14. Wake up stiff in the morning
15. Feel as if your body lacks solidity, substance
16. Weak muscles
17. Lack of fitness
18. Feel physically fragile, fear of getting bumped or jostled
19. Pain in bones, especially in lower back
20. Joint tenderness or inflammation

21. Tendency to cramps in legs, feet or toes, especially at night
22. Extreme fatigue
23. Heart palpitations
24. Experience hot flashes
25. Brittle or soft fingernails
26. Premature gray hair
27. Diet high in salt
28. Unusually lean, low body fat
29. Immoderate exercise (with second-degree amenorrhea, called athletic amenorrhea)
30. Being over 50
31. Nulliparity (no children, for women)
32. History of anorexia nervosa, overdieting, bulimia or simply being thin
33. Early (before age 45) menopause
34. Stooped posture, forward bending of spine (Dowager's hump)
35. Transparent skin
36. Declining height (averages 1.5 inches every 10 years after menopause; loss of .5 to 1 inch in a year is considered diagnostic)
37. Low peak bone mass in early adulthood, or small, fine bones
38. Prolonged immobility due to paralysis or illness
39. Fractures, especially vertebral crush, wrists or forearms and hips
40. High-protein diet, especially meat-based rather than vegetable- and whole grain-based
41. Drinking fluoridated water
42. Genetic predisposition, especially: fair skinned, small boned, family history (especially of Osteogenesis Imperfecta, a rare condition), northern European or Asian extraction, female gender

Diseases such as:

43. Chronic renal (kidney) disease, including kidney stones
44. Chronic liver disease
45. Hypogonadism (male or female sex organs don't produce high enough sex hormone levels)
46. Hyperthyroidism (thyrotoxicosis)
47. Adrenal overactivity (Cushing's syndrome)
48. Parathyroid overactivity (called hyperparathyroidism)
49. Other endocrine disease, including thyrotoxicosis
50. Rheumatoid arthritis
51. Chronic lung disease
52. Some forms of cancer, especially myeloma
53. Rickets

Have had surgical procedures such as:

54. Removal of ovaries
55. Removal of part or all of stomach or intestine
56. Hysterectomy
57. Prostatectomy
58. Gall bladder dysfunction or removal

Taking particular drugs, especially:

59. Anticonvulsants
60. Corticosteroids (used for asthma or rheumatoid arthritis)
61. Anticholinergics
62. Certain diuretics (loop diuretics, i.e., furosemide; Lasix and thiazides)
63. Anticoagulants (such as heparin or coumadin)
64. Antibiotics, especially tetracycline
65. Too high a dose of thyroid hormone replacement
66. Antacids containing aluminum

67. Phenothiazine derivatives
68. Lithium
69. Certain cancer chemotherapy medications
70. Radiation exposure, including from medical treatment

Other factors include:

71. Estrogen deficient (postmenopausal or surgical menopause)
72. Testosterone deficient (for men)
73. Inadequate dietary calcium
74. Insufficient exposure to sunshine, resulting in inadequate levels of Vitamin D
75. Smoke cigarettes
76. Lack exercise, a sedentary lifestyle
77. Ingest caffeine, especially excessive caffeine intake
78. Ingest alcohol

Experience related conditions such as:

79. Allergies
80. Frequent colds and infections
81. Gallstones or kidney stones
82. Cold sores or Herpes
83. Mitral valve insufficiency or prolapse
84. Arthritic or bony spurs

Any one of the above factors is sufficient to signal risk of osteoporosis; the higher the score, the greater the risk.

Now that you've checked these warning signs against your own experience, you may feel concerned that you're losing your bones. Maybe that's true. But please, remember the situation is not hopeless. You do not have to sit passively while you turn into a jellyfish!

How do I know? For one thing, you are assessing your situation now, and the sooner you become aware of it, the easier it will be to do something effective about it. And I know there are effective choices because I recovered my bones, and so have many others.

Our collective experiences indicate that the health or disease of bones is linked to that of the whole body, which is designed to maintain homeostasis, or a balanced state of health. From this perspective, osteoporosis can be seen as a solution: an attempt by the body to maintain this life-giving balance in the face of some formidable challenges. For this reason, we have concluded that "bones want to be healthy" and will move into a more healthy state whenever possible.

The rest of this book details what we learned.

ENDNOTES

1. Osteoporosis and Related Bone Diseases National Resource Center, National Osteoporosis Foundation, National Institutes of Health, Washington, D.C., June 1996 and July 1997, p. 1.
2. James Balch, M.D., and Phyllis A. Balch, C.N.C. Prescription for Nutritional Healing, Second Edition, Avery, Garden City, N.J., 1997., p. 413.
3. From an article entitled "Science Matters", *Ukiah Daily Journal*, Sun. Mar. 30, 1997, p. A–11.
4. Wyeth-Ayerst Laboratories advertisement, *USA Weekend* magazine, Sept. 26-28, 1997, p. 11.
5. Prempro ad, by Wyeth-Ayerst Labs, *USA Weekend*, Sept. 19–21, 1997, pp. 24–5.
6. Gail Sheehy. *New Passages, Mapping Your Life across Time*, Random House, New York, 1995, p. 200.
7. Clare Dover. *Osteoporosis*, Ward Lock in conjunction with the National Osteoporosis Society, London, England, 1994, p. 11.
8. Available: http://www.osteoporosis.org.au

9. Available: http://www.osteo.newsgallup.htm

10. Royal Lee. *Therapeutic Food Manual*, No publication date.

11. Royal Lee, D.D.S. Ibid.

12. Bernard Jensen and Mark Anderson. *Empty Harvest, Understanding the Link between Our Food, Our Immunity, and Our Planet*. Avery Publishing Group, Inc., Garden City Park, New York, 1990, pp. 10, 24, 47.

13. John Lee, M.D. *Natural Progesterone, The Multiple Roles of a Remarkable Hormone*, BLL Publishing, Sebastopol, Ca., 1993, p. 37.

14. Sources include: The National Osteoporosis Foundation; The Journal of the American Dietetic Association; The Johns Hopkins Medical Newsletter; The Mount Sinai Journal of Medicine; The Medical Data Exchange (MDX); "Healthwatch" in *NurseWeek*, Mae Tinklenberg, MS, RN, June 24, 1966; "Bone Up to Prevent Osteoporosis" in the Women's Health section of *Energy Times*, Jan. 1997, p. 18; and John Lee, M.D.'s *Natural Progesterone*.

15. Valerie Peck, M.D. "Depression-osteoporosis link found", *Ukiah Daily Journal*, March 30, 1997, p. A-11.

~~~ CHAPTER TWO

When Bad Bones Happen to Good People

Which Good People Are Most Likely to Get Bad Bones?

How is it that some people have more risk of their bones becoming porous and osteoporotic than others? After all, every human body is designed to have 206 bones, and every human body is designed the same way. Too, every human's bones are composed of the same three parts described before: the tough, outer layer; a spongy, middle layer; and a center containing marrow. Isn't it odd that osteoporosis is not an "equal opportunity" disease? For example, if it's true, as studies suggest, that bone mass peaks by age 30 to 35 and declines thereafter, and that women typically undergo a 30 to 40 percent bone loss between ages 50 and 70, wouldn't it follow that every woman would be stooped over and unable to function by her seventh decade?

The answer to that last question is undeniably "no"! And, one of the first factors that shows up to separate the lucky from the unlucky, of all things, is race! British author Clare Dover explains:

> When human life first emerged in the Rift Valley of Africa 200,000 years ago, we came with skeletons which were heavy and dense and extremely powerful. However, as our ancestors migrated, moving up the globe into higher latitudes,

17

genetic changes took place which caused a deterioration in the quality of the human skeleton. The European and other lighter skinned races became lighter boned...black women of African descent do not get osteoporosis with anything like the severity of white women. They are the inheritors of the original human skeleton...in adolescence black children are laying down an additional 34 percent of bone, [while] white children are undergoing an average 11 percent increase.[1]

Naturopathic physician Peter D'Adamo has studied this phenomenon in depth as he has worked to find the links between blood type and the incidence of certain diseases. He, too, saw this pattern:

The movement of the early humans to less temperate climates created lighter skins, less massive bone structures, and straighter hair. Nature, over time, reacclimated them to the regions of the earth they inhabited. People moved northward, so light skin developed, which was better protected against frostbite than dark skin. Lighter skin was also better able to metabolize vitamin D in a land of shorter days and longer nights.[2]

Another factor crucial to whether or not someone will develop osteoporosis is how much bone mass they developed before the menopausal decade. Studies have shown that

Total bone calcium in women increases from about 25 grams at birth to about 390 grams by age 10, requiring an average retention of 100 milligrams of calcium per day during childhood (one gram is about 1/30th of an ounce). With adolescence bone calcium more than doubles, reaching 800–1000 grams by age 18–20. At the peak of adolescent growth, bones require daily retention of 350–400 mgms. of calcium.[3]

Then, at around age 30 to 35, both men and women begin to lose bone at the slow rate of "about .3–.5% per year." In the 5 to 10 years after menopause, women lose about

> 15% of their total skeletal mass...Current medical research suggests that bone loss is going to occur after age 40, regardless of what we do...If we can achieve the greatest amount of bone strength and density in the years between 25 to 40, then our bones can afford to lose some density with age without risking fracture or disintegration.[4]

As Dover points out, by the time fractures actually occur,

> the skeleton may have lost 30 percent of the calcium that should be its source of strength...When several vertebrae have collapsed, there is a loss of height because of the shortening and compression of the spine. This reduces the capacity of the chest and abdominal cavities and interferes with the action of the heart, lungs, stomach and bladder and can cause difficulties in breathing, hiatus hernia and incontinence. The catalogue of suffering extends far beyond broken bones.[5]

These studies seem to be saying that to prevent problems in the later phases of life, one must have had the forethought, first of all, to have been born dark skinned, and secondly, to have made really strong bones as a child and adolescent! Since it's too late for all of us to change the first and too late for most of us to change the latter, what can be done? Is the situation really that hopeless? That is not my experience, nor is it the experience of the people who have addressed the roots of their bone weaknesses, as we shall see.

Your Bone Bank

The analogy of a bone bank is useful to better understand what happens in osteoporosis. It's like each person has a bone bank account opened during fetal life. Deposits are made and maintained in this account at a brisk pace during childhood and adolescence when growth is rapid. Everyone can not only make deposits, but also withdrawals. In osteoporosis, for whatever reason or reasons, withdrawals occur at a far more rapid rate than deposits. If the account had plenty to draw on in the first place, the symptoms of osteoporosis won't show up for quite a while. But if the account had little surplus to begin with, any slight increase in withdrawals can throw it over the edge. In this respect, osteoporosis can be considered to be a symptom of bone bankruptcy!

Bone bank deposits are made, kept and withdrawn through a cycle of metabolism that continuously forms, maintains and breaks down bones. If you are dark skinned, you have an apparent genetic advantage in that you have greater deposits in your bone bank to begin with, so that when withdrawals are made, you have farther to go before reaching a danger point. Also, the sum total of these deposits is usually greater in adult men than they are in adult women on average. In part, this is because men lay down thicker bones during their bone-building phase, and also because women make massive bone bank withdrawals to sustain pregnancy and lactation. Nonetheless, no matter what your genetic background, imbalances in any one or more of these three phases of the cycle can produce osteoporosis.

You already have a bone bank account, and your body has been making deposits, holding resources and making withdrawals all your life. No matter what the current state of your account, the Six-Point Plan for Perfect Bones will give you the information you need to learn to manage this bodily bank account in the same way you'd learn to manage any other investment, such as real estate, a retirement fund or a stock or bond. In fact, thinking of managing your bone bank so that you'll have sufficient resources for your retirement years is both an accurate parallel and a healthy goal. To accomplish this, you only need consider six basic points.

The Six-Point Plan and Your Bone Bank

The components of the six-point plan are

1. Healthy Connective Tissue
2. Sufficient Minerals and Their Vitamin Helpers
3. Essential Fatty Acids and the Ability to Metabolize Them
4. A Balanced Hormonal System
5. Proper Digestive, Eliminative and Muscular Activity
6. A Clean Environment and Healthy Immune System

(These are first summarized below, then presented, each in its own chapter, in Part Two.)

Every one of the six points of the plan for perfect bones is essential to bone health. Each plays a crucial role in the cycle of making bone bank deposits, helping maintain them, or permitting withdrawals so the body can support cell activities everywhere. In turn, each is central to the health of the entire body.

The first two of the six points deal with deposits. Instead of carrying in dollars and cents like in a monetary bank account, cells called osteoblasts transport deposits of collagen (connective tissue) and minerals. The connective tissue forms little fibrous beams that hold their payload of mineral deposits in beautiful crystals called calcium apatite that are engineered like tiny bridges. In a bank, these would be made of steel and called safe deposit boxes. In bone, they are collagen structures, connective tissues made of various proteins. A key to perfecting your bones, then, is to make substantial deposits of all the various components of collagen (point one) and the minerals (point two) needed to form these crystal bone bridges. This is possible because the skeleton repairs itself with fresh calcium atoms every three months. In fact, 98 percent of the body's atoms are exchanged for new ones every year. A key to healing, then, is to make those atoms top-quality food so it can repair and express optimum health.[6]

The role of getting these deposits to the bank falls to the food group known as oils, or essential fatty acids (point three). They function like an armored vehicle that safely delivers deposits to the bank. Without these carriers, materials bones need are left by the metabolic wayside, where they can eventually turn into roadblocks for other bodily processes. To get them out of the way, the body may put them in other tissues, causing soft, pliable tissues such as eardrums or the inside of arteries to harden. Or, it may gather the minerals together to eliminate them, in the process forming stones in the gall bladder or kidneys.

The rate of these activities, whether to increase, hold, or withdraw deposits, is governed by hormones (point four). Pituitary, thyroid and parathyroid, adrenal, and gonadal hormones provide this direction in concert. For example, the cells that make bone bank withdrawals, called osteoclasts, have the role of reabsorbing and removing bone that needs repair. Far from being bad guys, these cells help keep bone healthy. They recognize places in need of mending, and they tear away the less than healthy bone. That makes room for osteoblasts to put new deposits in and restore health. They are stimulated to carry out this function by parathyroid hormone, and inhibited from making withdrawals by the thyroid hormone calcitonin. In women, these bone bank withdrawals are carried out at a much more rapid rate after the hormonal changes of menopause, but by about the 65th year, the rate for men and women is the same.

These glandular hormone factories even cooperate; they pick up the slack for each other when necessary. However, if one of the hormone factories stops putting out its contribution, another one can only substitute for a while, and then it, too, becomes exhausted.

If nothing is done to correct the imbalance, the whole house of cards can eventually come tumbling down into a state of total bone bankruptcy.

The process of absorption (point five) determines what materials are made available to run these metabolic activities. The whole operation has to be kept moving along, with fresh supplies brought in and old materials no longer needed eliminated as quickly as possible. If the process should bog down anywhere, the entire flow can back up, eventually shutting down everything.

The focus of point six is protecting this life-giving cycle of depositing, storing and withdrawing. Thieves, robbers and embezzlers, in the form of toxins, allergic reactions, and infections, skulk about, waiting to carry out their nefarious activities. The body must maintain the integrity of the bone crystals and their supporting structures and hold bones' mineral treasure in the face of such attacks. Bone banks are vulnerable to robbery of their precious contents.

Some bone robbers arrive in the form of viruses, parasites or bacteria that emit toxins which render the bone 'deposit boxes' incapable of holding their priceless treasure. Others create emergencies in other parts of the body, causing the hormones' directors to send messages to release bones' deposits and make their riches available to fight invasion elsewhere. These messengers might say, for example, "Never mind that your bones need these minerals to maintain their strength. Your heart needs them much more right now to keep beating, and if your heart doesn't beat, there's no reason to worry about your bones. Healthy heart contractions are much more important than healthy bones!"

The Collective Cost

The personal cost of osteoporosis begins with having to live what life you have fearing that if you sneeze, or pick up a bag of groceries, or get jostled in a crowd, you'll fracture a bone. Once diagnosed, you know you face a life of declining health, bone fractures, unrelenting pain and death. But this profound suffering is not the only kind of cost. What is the cost to society when bad bones happen to good people?

The statistics are staggering: osteoporosis is responsible for over 1 million fractures a year in men and women over the age of 45—with many of these fractures resulting in long-term debilitation and unrelenting pain. In fact, one of every two women older than age 50 will suffer an osteoporosis-related fracture during her lifetime![7] In the United States, some 40,000 osteoporosis victims annually die within six months of their fractures. Fifty percent of all people who experience osteoporosis-related hip fractures never regain the ability to walk independently. Fifty percent also end up in nursing homes following a hip fracture. Indeed, more women will die from complications of osteoporosis than die from breast and cervical cancer and heart disease together! In fact, the World Health Organization lists osteoporosis as the second largest world health problem next to cardiovascular disease. And the University of Colorado is campaigning to have osteoporosis defined as a pediatric-onset disease!

A full one-third of all American women will develop osteoporosis severe enough to cause a fracture, while it is estimated that at age 60, a man has a 25 percent chance of breaking a hip or vertebra during his life. And, says Eric S. Orwoll, M.D., more men than women die after a hip fracture![8] Indeed, "one in every 8 men over age 50 will have an osteoporosis-related fracture. Each year, 80,000 men suffer a hip fracture and one-third of them die within a year."[9] In 1985, the national cost of these osteoporosis fractures was estimated to be $7 billion a year![10]

In the United Kingdom, the Royal College of Physicians found that patients with hip fractures occupied 20 percent of orthopedic beds, and that 80 percent of these were women over 65 years old.[11] In fact, the Royal College estimates that one in four women over 70 and one in 20 men have osteoporosis and will sustain a fracture related to it. And hip fractures lead to fatal complications in 12 to 20% of cases! "Each year doctors in the UK see more than 60,000 hip fractures, 50,000 wrist fractures, 40,000 spinal fractures and about 50,000 other fractures related to osteoporosis."[12] The United Kingdom spends only 61 million pounds on hormone replacement therapy, but problems caused by osteoporosis cost the Health Service more than one billion pounds a year![13]

In Canada, the cost of treating femoral fractures alone exceeds $400 million per year. By 2010, the estimated cost of osteoporosis to Canada's health care system will be *one billion dollars annually!*

Measuring the cost of osteoporosis by examining femoral fracture statistics reveals only part of the cost. The leading cause of death for women in America is reported to be heart disease, which at first may seem unrelated to osteoporosis. But the calcium the heart needs to continue beating, when not available from the diet, is borrowed from bones. Once the bones are bankrupt of their calcium treasures (osteoporotic), heart failure is not far behind. Yet these deaths are reported as heart failure, not as end-stage osteoporosis, a procedure which hides costs that could prove to be 10 times more than those calculated using hip fracture statistics.

In America, death from osteoporosis is reported to be the 12th leading cause of mortality. Only those who die due to complications from bone fractures and falls are counted in that number. Still, osteoporosis is estimated to cost the nation *$3.8 billion.*[14] And, it will get worse! Why?

To the 25 million people currently suffering from osteoporosis in the U.S. are now being added 20 million more baby boomers entering menopause before the turn of the century. Another way of saying this is that baby boomers are currently turning 50 at the rate of nine per second and that there are 76 million of them.[15] Demographers point out that by the year 2030, 69 million of us will be 65 or older, with 9 million being 85 or older. Sixty years from now, the number of people at risk for osteoporosis is expected to triple, in other words, to reach 135 million!

Eighty percent of those affected by osteoporosis are women (according to The National Osteoporosis Foundation), the usual caregivers not only of children, but of the frail and elderly. There will be fewer and fewer able-bodied caregivers for a population whose average age is getting older and older. The Chronic Care Consortium estimates that there are already some 99 million people in the U.S. today with chronic health conditions, with the number expected to grow to 150 million by the year 2030. Clearly, a health crisis of societal proportions due to osteoporosis is on the horizon. Society simply does not have the resources to cope with this enormous problem.

But the cost of bad bones is not limited to middle-aged people. Two potentially life-threatening conditions in pregnancy have been shown to be pre-osteoporotic; in other words, to exist prior to bone bankruptcy. They are pregnancy-induced hypertension (high blood pressure) and pre-eclampsia, a toxic state in pregnancy that can lead to convulsions, coma and death. These maladies affect 1 in 7 pregnant women, and are the leading cause of Cesarean-sections, pre-term births and low-birth-weight babies, costing society *billions* of dollars. But that's just the beginning! To that figure must be added the total cost of care for premature infants in the United States, which is *$20–40 billion per year*. And then to that must be added the cost of hospital care of a low birth-weight baby, which can run *$7000 per day*, or as much as *half a million dollars per infant!*[16]

Not included in these costs is any amount for dental problems. It is unknown at this time how many dental syndromes such as cavities, teeth cracking, shattering, wearing down or becoming loose in their sockets are the result of the body borrowing their calcium. Nor do these figures include any estimate of the cost of various immunologic disturbances.

In summary, a conservative estimate by the National Institute of Health of the social cost in the United States alone (excluding statistics for dental problems, pregnancy and low-birth-weight babies, and heart problems) is $10 billion annually, a cost that is expected to double over 30 years![17]

Clearly something must be done. But is help available? Let's turn first to the place most people turn when they have a health problem: their local physician.

ENDNOTES

1. Clare Dover. Ibid., p. 13.
2. Peter D'Adamo. *Eat Right For Your Type*, Riverhead/Putnam, New York, 1996, p. 8.
3. "Calcium, Beneficial to Bones and More" in *Healthy Cell News*, Spring/Summer 1996, p. 17.
4. "Calcium, Beneficial to Bones and More," Ibid., p. 17.
5. Clare Dover. Ibid., pp. 8, 10.
6. D. A. Versendaal, D.C., Ph.D., Author's Interview.
7. Lisa Lanucci. "Bone Power," in *Energy Times*, May 1997, p. 59.
8. Jean Carper. "Calcium: Not for women only," in *U.S.A. Weekend*, March 27–29, p. 15.
9. National Osteoporosis Foundation. "Men with Osteoporosis, in their own words." National Osteoporosis Foundation, Washington, D.C., 1997.
10. Available at: medlineplus.nlm.nih.gov/medlineplus/osteoporosis.html
11. Clare Dover., Ibid., p. 8.
12. Clare Dover. Ibid., p. 36.
13. Clare Dover. Ibid., p. 33.
14. Balch and Balch, Ibid., p. 413.
15. Horace B. Deets, "A.A.R.P.'s Realignment" in AARP Perspectives, *Modern Maturity*, Nov–Dec. 1997, p. 1.

16. Journal of the American Medical Association Reports: Calcium During Pregnancy Could Save Lives. Available at http://www.kidsource.com/kidsource/content/news/calcium.4.9.html
See also http://wwwsenate.gov/~dpc/sr/sr-o1.html
17. Available: www.columbia.net/consumer/datafile/osteo.html, no date.

CHAPTER THREE

Bones Are Bones:
The Western Medical Paradigm

Ask for a description of the typical osteoporosis sufferer, and you'd likely get a list with words like middle aged or old woman, dowager's hump, slow moving, tired looking, hunched over, walks with a cane or walker, weak, poor muscle tone, resigned attitude, depressed, downcast, etc. Yet here came Carol Gieg to our first meeting, bouncing down the steps on a hot August afternoon. Her short shorts and a halter top revealed not an ounce of fat anywhere, and the perfect muscle development of a world class woman athlete. At 5 feet 5 inches tall and 105 pounds, on the cusp of turning 40, she looked to be in enviable physical shape.

As we settled into chairs in my office and began to talk, I soon discovered how wrong this impression was. Her first bone fracture occurred at age nine, she revealed. This was followed by a greenstick fracture and a broken foot at age twelve, a dislocated shoulder at age seventeen and a broken hand at twenty-three, facts she put off to being so active. But she'd also had only one period, at age sixteen, and none after that. By twenty-one, she went in quest of normalizing this situation. Her first physician at the University of California in San Francisco was just beginning research on the links between fat-estrogen levels and osteoporosis. He conducted a variety of tests, then told her not to worry. The next year, during a marathon race, she heard her hip break.

Still recovering, she next turned to a second physician who put her on crutches, thinking it would rest her bones. It was a big mistake, she said, for her condition worsened.

A third physician put her on some hormones, including FSH (follicle stimulating hormone). A fourth one, a nephrologist (kidney specialist) studying the metabolic process in the kidney, started her on estrogen. He also took a punch biopsy of the bone in her hip and sent it off to a fifth one, a University of Kentucky specialist. His diagnosis came back: osteogenesis imperfecta tarda, a congenital bone disease causing the bones to fracture easily, for which there is little medical science can do. Feeling hopeless, she gave up trying to get better and just tried to live with it.

Eventually the pain and discomfort became too much, however. This time she turned to alternative practitioners and a combination of massage, chiropractic and a macrobiotic diet began to ease the pain. Still, she was very fragile physically. Attending the University of California at Berkeley where she was working on dual masters degrees in Social Work and Public Health, she kept a motorized scooter at each end of her commute train, where she would ride to school and park next to the building where her classes were located. No one ever knew her condition. Then she heard about the use of Calcitonin injections for Paget's disease (chronic inflammation of the bones with thickening and distortion, also known as *osteitis deformans*).

Turning now to a sixth physician, she began Calcitonin injections, only to become so sick to her stomach after each one that despite her desire to regain her bone health, she eventually threw the drug away.

Her seventh doctor was one she met during her work at a Bay Area children's hospital. She had now endured pain for 10 years. He told her unequivocally, "You have to gain some weight!" Conducting some lab tests, he told her immune function lab results were lower than those of a person with AIDS! Realizing the truth in what he was saying, she gave up macrobiotics, concluding that it hadn't helped, except that it had given her hope.

Then she heard of an eighth physician at the University of Worster in Massachusetts and called him on the phone. He kindly consented to review her records, by now a pile of documents several inches thick. He called her back early in the morning on July 4th and said, "You don't have OI (osteogenesis imperfecta); that was not a correct analysis and the bone sample they took was too small to make a correct conclusion. You have severe osteoporosis." And he never sent a bill.

Relieved, frustrated and confused, she widened her search and turned up a ninth physician in California specializing in using natural progesterone (see Part Two, Chapter 9). She began to use ProGest Cream made from Mexican yams instead of Premarin and Provera (synthetic chemicals that mimic natural hormones, see *Medical Treatment Approaches* below). And she took a course in meditation and one in restorative yoga. She learned to breathe into the pain and relax deep muscle tissues that were constantly tense, and finally began to gain some pain relief.

She next visited a tenth physician, a woman who gave her phytoestrogens and some herbs. That was followed with an eleventh physician, an endocrinologist who wanted to try kick starting her body's own estrogen production. She stopped all hormones, even avoiding the natural estrogens in soy products. By the second month she had lost breast mass, had dark circles under her eyes and felt awful. Unwilling to continue like this, she resumed ProGest cream in a 10% concentration. In the first four years on ProGest cream, bone density studies showed a slight increase in bone mass. Then during the fifth year in which she was very job-stressed she lost all the bone she had gained. Her last bone density study, at the Osteoporosis and Related Bone Diseases National Resource Center, revealed the same results: that her bone age was that of a 76-year-old woman![1]

With such a history, I could see why she was so weary of searching. As a social worker who has spent her adult life help-ing people, she definitely qualified as a good person to whom bad things had happened!

The Medical Paradigm and Your Bones

Carol's ordeal is repeated thousands of times over every day as suf-ferers search for answers. Their experiences demonstrate some of the basic principles that underlie current medical thinking about osteoporosis:

1. that everybody's bones are the same;
2. that everybody's osteoporosis is the same;
3. that everybody's osteoporosis can be treated the same way;
4. that appropriate treatment addresses symptoms rather than causes;
5. that such treatment consists of administering drugs until body parts are surgically replaced; and
6. that there is no cure.

These principles are fundamental to a tradition of thought about disease that medical historian Harris Coulter, in his three-volume work *Divided Legacy*, calls the "Rational School". Visible in medical thought for 2000 years, the rational school uses logical analysis rather than observation and experience as the source of knowlege and studies disease entities rather than growth. It clas-sifies common symptoms into disease entities, and once a hypoth-esis of causation is established, bases its treatment approach on chemical (drugs) or mechanistic (surgery) approaches.[2]

Most treatment for osteoporosis, therefore, consists of admin-istering one or more synthetic chemicals to affect the course of the disease. Since the body operates on the principle that "for every action there is an equal and opposite reaction," these chemicals have both a therapeutic effect and side effects, meaning results other than the therapeutic ones. For example, if a drug stimulates the body, it eventually will produce a letdown. The person first feels like they're getting better, but then they crash somehow or other.

With regard to osteoporosis, Alan Gaby, M.D., President-elect of the American Holistic Medical Association, summarizes the current medical viewpoint:

> Conventional medical opinion is that osteoporosis is a relentless process that cannot be reversed and that the best we can hope for is to slow down the rate of bone loss.[3]

Dr. John Lee adds, "Present osteoporosis management emphasizes prevention rather than cure since true reversal has proven unobtainable by conventional methods."[4]

Given that these beliefs underlie the medical options that will be offered to osteoporosis sufferers, let us now look at these components more closely.

Medical Diagnosis of Osteoporosis

Bone loss used to be diagnosed with x-rays, which don't show bone loss until 25 to 40%, even 50% of the skeleton has been depleted.[5] The primary tests now used to diagnose osteoporosis are bone mineral density studies (BMD). These use a radioactive photon beam; bone with greater mineral content absorbs more photons. Single photon tests usually check the wrist or heel bones. Dual photon tests (DPA) can check the hip or spine. The newer "DEXA", which is the abbreviation for dual x-ray absorptiometry test, uses x-rays.

"DEXA" does not truly measure bone mineral density as such, but rather measures the amount of calcium, which is a surrogate marker for bone density, and is therefore less accurate, particularly in elderly patients. Therefore, "bone mineral density deviations are diagnostic guidelines, not treatment thresholds."[6] The medical community considers the DPA and DEXA tests to be state of the art for measuring bone loss.

The tests require expensive equipment that is unavailable in many areas. Typically, two measurements are taken a year apart to measure the rate of bone loss, a test that costs around $200 each, and may or may not be covered by insurance.

If you are going to use such a test to attempt to follow your state of bone health or the effectiveness of a treatment for osteoporosis, Dr. John Lee recommends using the lumbar vertebrae (the bones in your lower spine) rather than the usual trabecular bone (the spongy interior portion of the bone that's most susceptible to osteoporosis). That's because these bones are "relatively large and uniform, the test results are generally more clinically accurate."

He also advises that when having serial tests, "different techniques give slightly different results and, therefore, comparisons of test results using different techniques are not as good as using the same technique throughout. Further, it is wise to use the same equipment in the same testing facility, if possible."[7]

However, bone mineral density test results do not correlate directly with the health of bone. "Ideally," states J. C. Prior of the Division of Endocrinology and Metabolism at the University of British Columbia, the results of such tests "should be shown to correlate with the ashed mineral content of the bone, to parallel the tensile strength of bone, and predict the fracture frequency. None of the reported measurements can yet meet all these criteria."[8]

Indeed, according to J. E. Compston, Dept. of Medicine, University of Cambridge, some studies report that large increases in bone mass as seen in bone mineral density studies may actually be associated with a *reduced* bone strength and *unchanged or increasing* fracture rates! In fact, recent studies "indicate that fracture prevention is not necessarily associated with increase in bone density."[9] Truly healthy bones are not only dense, they are also flexible, supple and strong as a result of healthy microarchitecture. BMD tests don't measure these characteristics, which correlate more with fracture rates than density. Bones that appear to be dense can actually be unhealthy—brittle, rigid and prone to breakage. In fact, some medical treatments currently prescribed to treat osteoporosis cause bones to become more dense, therefore appearing healthy in BMD measurements, but actually become more dense and *brittle*, and therefore more prone to fracture. To be truly healthy, bones must be both supple and dense.

Another disadvantage of relying on BMD tests to determine bone health is that they only measure the density of one bone. But bones can vary in density from one to another. Also, calcium deposits may be thicker in one area, causing the machine to produce a higher density reading than is truly correct. Additionally, test results are compared to the peak bone density of typical premenopausal women, not women in the same age group, thus discounting normal differences associated with age groups.

That's why some doctors are now using tests to measure the levels of some of the by-products of bone breakdown in the urine. These tests have several advantages: they might uncover bone loss in its earlier stages; they carry no risk of exposure to x-rays or photons; and they are far less expensive than DPA or DEXA. However, results can vary by up to 40 or even 50% from one day to the next![10] And, higher calcium excretion does *not* mean the calcium is being taken from the bone. For example, the body could be dumping calcium in conjunction with a high protein intake where the body is attempting to balance phosphorus.

Their problem at this point is that normal lab values for people of different ages are not known, leaving the interpretation of results a matter of opinion. Also, a great deal depends on when in the course of bone breakdown the tests are taken: urinary calcium is increased in the initial phases of bone depletion, normal later, and low when the bone bank calcium deposits are drained.

When doctors want to know the condition of different areas of bone, they may order a bone scan, which requires being injected with a radioactive dye.

Medical Treatment Approaches

Once the diagnosis is decided upon, what are the medical treatment options for osteoporosis? Current treatments consist of administering one or more synthetic chemicals which block the body's ability to make bone bank account withdrawals. As J. E. Compston, of the Department of Medicine, University of Cambridge, summarizes, "Nearly all treatments available are antiresorptive."

Because each option is a drug, it produces two reactions: a therapeutic effect and side effects. The long-term effects of new drugs are not yet known. This fact could prove to have major significance in osteoporosis. If bone resorption is affected in some way, healthy bone usually compensates with a change in the amount of new bone formed. Thus it is theoretically possible that by reducing bone resorption, these drugs may actually lower the rate of new bone formation, ultimately increasing the problem they were designed to treat.

Below are listed the prescription drugs currently available, how they act to treat osteoporosis sufferers, and how each one works relative to the bone bank metabolic cycle of depositing, maintaining and withdrawing. All are purported to slow down the course of the disease, not cure it.

ERT (Estrogen Replacement Therapy) (for women). The original medical approach to osteoporosis was estrogen replacement therapy (see Part Two, Chapter 9). Currently doctors in the U.S. prescribe $840 million worth of estrogen supplements.[11] ERT for postmenopausal women is based on the observation that bone bank withdrawals are made at a much more rapid rate when levels of estrogen are low. Apparently low estrogen levels stimulate bone bank withdrawals: osteoclast bone cells speed up the rate at which they are reabsorbing bone (withdrawing from the bone bank). The idea is that increasing estrogen levels will slow this rapid breakdown rate.

The studies of ERT's effect on bone were originally conducted on women who were already severely osteoporotic, and ERT's effect on bone was measured by a decreased incidence of fractures. *The role of estrogen in actually preventing bone loss before it occurs has not been determined, although it is widely prescribed for that purpose.* John Lee, M.D., points out that the positive results seen on the bones of women who were already severely osteoporotic "fades in 5 years or so and, thereafter, bone loss continues at the same pace as in those women not using estrogen."[12]

Nonetheless, 1 in 5 menopausal women uses estrogen replacement therapy today. A recent report in *Women's Health News* observes: "Contrary to what hormone supplement manufacturers would like you to believe, the widely advertised health benefits of lower heart disease and osteoporosis risk with HRT [hormone replacement therapy] are not standing up to long-term scrutiny."[13] To summarize: estrogen replacement therapy does not help bone loss which has already occurred; however, it does slow the rate of bone loss, from 5% on average to 1% for women taking it in the first 5 years after menopause.

Premarin is one such product commonly used. In fact, it accounts for about 90% of the prescriptions for estrogen replacement ($672 million per year). States William Campbell Douglass, M.D.: "Unfortunately Premarin does NOT contain the same estrogen your body produces. [Premarin is made from horse's urine and contains over 49 different horse estrogens, none of which is naturally found in humans.[14]] As a result, Premarin's effects on osteoporosis have been disappointing. What's worse, Premarin has a whole host of negative side effects, including physical addiction . . . and an increased risk of breast cancer!"[15]

A 1995 study reported in *The New England Journal of Medicine* underscores Dr. Douglass' opinion. Involving 121,790 women who used synthetic estrogens and progestins to offset symptoms of menopause, it found that these women also increased their chance of developing breast cancer by up to 40% by taking these synthetic chemicals more than 5 years!

Other side effects may include nausea, bloating, stomach cramping, vomiting, headache, breast tenderness and enlargement, water retention and edema, mood changes, vaginal bleeding, high blood pressure, and increased risk of uterine cancer.[16] Estrogen therapy has also been found to promote gallstones, rare liver tumors, and blood clotting. It is contraindicated in the presence of obesity, varicose veins, hyperlipidemias, fibrocystic breast disease, a history of breast cancer, endometrial cancer or uterine cancer, clotting disorders, or thromboembolism, liver disease, hypertension, smoking, and heart disease.

In addition to the side effects, some women refuse to take Premarin because its production causes great suffering to mares. They are first impregnated and then hooked up to catheter-type devices to collect their urine, which is kept concentrated by keeping the mares dehydrated. Author and researcher John Robbins adds that they are also "forced to stand constantly on hard, cold, concrete floors, unable to take more than a couple steps, and are unable to lie down comfortably, for 7 of the 11 months of their pregnancy. Each year, 90,000 foals are 'disposed of' as an unwanted 'by-product'."[17]

Other researchers have noted that the same therapeutic effect produced by estrogen replacement therapy can be produced by supplementing with 3 mg. of boron per day so that the body can make its own estrogen. (See Part Two, Chapter 9.)

More recent arrivals on the market are the class of estrogen substitutes called "SERMS", which stands for "selective estrogen receptor modulator". They are "designer estrogens" (with the chemical name of raloxifene) which are hoped to mimic the good effects of estrogen, such as a lower risk of heart disease and stronger bones, while inhibiting any harmful effects, such as promoting uterine and breast cancer. One such product is Evista, marketed by Eli Lilly and Co., who paid for a study that claims there was a dramatic drop in the risk of breast cancer in women who took it. However, the study did not state what the absolute risk for breast cancer was in those particular women in the first place. Also, the drug had almost no effect on the kind of breast cancer most commonly developed by younger women and those with a genetic predisposition to it (estrogen-receptor-negative breast cancer). And, raloxifene increases the risk of serious blood clots.[18]

Progestins (again, usually for women, although used occasionally for men). More recently some doctors have begun to prescribe synthetic progestins. These are chemical imitations of the natural progesterone the body produces. The hormone progesterone has been shown to be far more important than estrogen for bone health: low progesterone levels mean reduced bone bank deposits. Dr. Lee states that a "lack of progesterone . . . causes a decrease in osteoblast-mediated new bone formation." Dr. Lee pioneered using natural progesterone creams for a wide variety of health problems (including pre-menstrual syndrome, fibrocystic breasts, fibroid tumors, ovarian cysts, endometriosis, endometrial carcinoma).

The state of affairs in which a woman's bodily progesterone levels are too low, he adds, are brought about by many factors, among them "nutritional deficiencies, stress, environmental xenoestrogens, toxins, follicular depletion, and of course, the hormonal imbalance induced by contraception pills composed of synthetic hormones."[19] He stresses that "progesterone deficiency and estrogen dominance" is the problem in most of the above-stated health problems, including osteoporosis. Does that mean it's best to go get a prescription for synthetic progestins? No, Dr. Lee states, "Provera, a progestin that differs from progesterone by a methyl group at carbon 6, has also been found to provide modest increases in bone density but lacks the full biological generality of natural progesterone and is not free of worrisome side effects. Additionally, its monthly costs are approximately 10 times that of transdermal progesterone."[20] He adds, "It is a mystery to me why synthetic progestins are recommended when the natural progesterone is available, cheaper and safer."[21]

One answer might be that some sources are claiming you don't get a 'therapeutic dose' using natural progesterone cream. In fact, however, the dose actually required is far lower when using the whole, naturally occuring complex.

Estrogen and Progestins in combination. In addition to the risks stated above for estrogen and progestin separately , side effects of the combination of drugs also include nausea, vomiting, pain, cramps, swelling or tenderness in the abdomen; yellowing of the skin and/or whites of the eyes; breast tenderness or enlargement; enlargement of benign tumors of the uterus; irregular bleeding or spotting; change in amount of cervical secretion, vaginal yeast infections; retention of excess fluid, which may worsen asthma, epilepsy, migraine, heart disease or kidney disease; a spotty dark-ening of the skin, particularly on the face; reddening of the skin; skin rashes; worsening of porphyria, headache, migraines, dizzi-ness, faintness or changes in vision (including intolerance to con-tact lenses); mental depression; involuntary muscle spasms; hair loss or abnormal hairiness; increase or decrease in weight; changes in the sex drive; possible changes in blood sugar.[22]

Although it is primarily used to restore the function of the vaginal mucosa and to increase libido in women, *testosterone* ther-apy has been used for both women and men with osteoporosis. It has been shown to increase bone density in those whose levels were too low and in some men with normal testosterone levels. The normal ovary produces some testosterone, and after meno-pause the adrenal glands provide some. "In women with testos-terone deficiency, addition of testosterone to an estrogen regimen may provide added protection against osteoporosis."[23] Tablets taken orally are composed of methyl-testosterone. Side effects include acne and hair growth, and, because testosterone is converted in the liver, is sometimes not tolerated in people with low liver functioning.

However, synthetic hormones, whether they are progestins, estrogen mimics, or testosterone substitutes, are chemical "look-alikes"—pictures of the hormones the body naturally produces. Because they substitute for real hormones, administration of any synthetic hormone actually can slow down or stop the body's own production, thus *lowering* the blood levels of the real hormone!

Editronate was approved because two studies showed it increased bone density and decreased new fractures in the spine for people who used it two years. However, a three-year study shows no difference in the rate of spinal fractures between those who took it and those who didn't. Even though it's been shown to produce denser bones, unfortunately, it also makes them softer (osteomalacia) rather than stronger.[24]

Biophosphonates are sold under the brand name Fosamax or generically as alendronate. Their action could be likened to having a chemical "stop payment" placed on some bone bank deposits so they can't be removed. They inhibit bone bank withdrawals by binding "tightly to hydroxyapatite crystals [the collagen and mineral crystal deposits that make up bone] and inhibit bone resorption."[25]

Like the studies that demonstrated the positive effects of hormone replacement therapy, the tests for biophosphonates were conducted on women with existing vertebral fractures. A University of California at San Francisco study showed that "among women with existing vertebral fractures alendronate is well tolerated and substantially reduces the incidence of vertebral and clinical fractures including the incidence of hip fractures by about half."

The long-term risks and side effects remain largely unknown because it has just been approved by the FDA and physicians are just beginning to prescribe it. Currently known side effects include nausea, esophageal and stomach irritation; abdominal pain;

bone, muscle and joint pain; headache; heartburn; altered sense of taste, and sometimes allergic reactions. The first generation of biophosphonates also had adverse effects on bone structure.[26]

Research on biophosphonates at the Department of Medicine, University of South Carolina, reports that these drugs inhibit osteoclastic (cells that resorb bone) bone resorption *at lower concentrations*. However, at higher concentrations they may *"inhibit mineralization and cause osteomalacia"*, a disease in which "the bones soften so that they become flexible and brittle and cause deformities. It is attended with rheumatic pains. The limbs, spine, thorax, and pelvis esp. are affected; anemia and signs of deficiency disease present; the patient becomes weak, and finally dies from exhaustion."[27] The research was reported by N. H. Bell and R. H. Johnson. They add that "bone formation is also reduced as a consequence of diminished bone resorption." In summary, because biophosphonates block bone resorption, they "come with the risk of actually impairing other important aspects of our health."[28]

Calcitonin (brand names are Calcimar, Cibacalcin). It is a synthetic chemical imitation of the calcitonin hormones produced by the thyroid gland. The natural hormone the body produces helps regulate blood levels of bone-building calcium and reduce the rate of bone bank withdrawals by inhibiting bone-destroying cells. The synthetic chemical version was formerly injected daily at a doctor's office; however, it is now available in a nasal spray (Miacalcin). It works as an antiresorptive agent and is for people whose bone density is already low but whose rate of bone turnover is high.

Calcitonin (the natural hormone produced by the body) is secreted by the thyroid gland. It inhibits the rate of bone bank withdrawals. "Calcitonin is a potent inhibitor of osteoclasts, the cells that cause bone resorption."[29] It is mentioned here because a chemical imitation of it has been produced (Calcimar) for osteoporosis. "When injected into humans," states John Lee, M.D., there is a brief period of new bone formation. With further sets of injections, the bone response becomes progressively less. When discontinued, the benefits gained are quickly lost."[30]

Nausea, rhinitis (inflammation of the nose with the nasal spray) and arthralgias (joint pain) are common side effects.[31] Other side effects, writes Alan Gaby, M.D., "include transient facial flushing, nausea with or without vomiting in about 10% of cases ... [and rarely] severe allergic reactions, including anaphylactic shock [an acute, life-threatening form of shock resulting from an allergic reaction], and one death due to anaphylaxis...." Dr. Gaby concludes, "At a cost of $7.50 per day (or more than $2,700 per year), calcitonin is probably the most expensive treatment for osteoporosis."[32]

Sodium fluoride is a chemical which has been put on teeth to reduce cavities and added to drinking water. It is now in development in a slow-release form for treatment of osteoporosis because it is purported to build new bone bank deposits, thus preventing fractures, when used in conjunction with calcium citrate. It is reported to be "the only widely tested drug that can stimulate new bone formation.

Apparently sodium fluoride makes bones more dense, so that they seem more healthy during bone density studies, but the resultant bone is less flexible, and therefore more likely to break. High doses of this drug were found to increase bone mass but to also impair bone strength."[33] Dr. John Lee underscores that fluoride "may slightly increase the x-ray appearance of bone mass but the resultant bone is of inferior quality and actually increases the risk of hip fracture" whether that fluoride is from osteoporosis therapy or fluoridated water. "Fluoride", he states "is a potent enzyme inhibitor and, in bone, causes pathologic changes leading to increased risk of fracture. Fluoride, in all forms including tooth pastes, should be avoided."[34] Additional side effects may include nausea, vomiting, diarrhea and leg pains. Alan Gaby, M.D., concurs: "Any potential benefit of fluoride treatment must be balanced against reports of serious side effects, including anemia, gastrointestinal symptoms, arthritis, and recurrent vomiting."[35] Indeed, states Michael Dobbins, D.C., "Fluoride is a highly toxic halogen."[36]

Minocycline. Another approach is the antibiotic minocycline. It has been shown to increase bone mass in laboratory animals and is now being tested on women.

Antibiotics kill off the natural flora of the body which help digest food and provide a natural protective barrier for the skin and G.I. tract. Antibiotics interfere with absorption of the various vitamins and minerals necessary for healthy bones. The natural intestinal flora also manufacture vitamin K, an essential helper in maintaining bone health. Their absence sets the stage for osteoporosis because the rate of bone bank withdrawals is dramatically increased as the body leaches calcium from the bone.

Also, since undigested food turns to poison in the body, antibiotics weaken the immune system's defenses. Immune and other cells cannot get the nutrition they need to function properly when their work load is greatly increased due to having to clean up so much undigested food. Use of antibiotics has meant trading short term help for long term problems.

Anti-depressants. Statistics have shown a correlation between depression and bone density, which is why drug companies encourage physicians to encourage their patients to take anti-depressants. Anti-depressants have a variety of side effects depending on the kind. Depression is also an indicator of hormone imbalances (see Part Two, Chapter 9).

Cytokines. Researchers are also looking at cytokines, which are naturally produced by the bone marrow. They are encoded proteins that control immune activity within the cell or at a distance. Their tiny immunologic messages can mediate or turn on or off immune system defenses. Cytokines can contribute to bone loss when several kinds act in concert.

Anabolic steroids are sometimes used for men who have osteoporosis because they help build bone and muscle mass. One drawback for women is that they masculinize. Women develop a mustache and deeper voice. They can also increase the risk of heart disease and can be toxic to the liver.

Additionally, a newly approved drug is *raloxifene*. It "acts like estrogen in the skeleton, guarding against bone loss, but blocks the growth-stimulating effects of estrogen in the breast and uterus, where hormone stimulation can lead to increased tumor development. Raloxifene is among the first compounds cultivated from a class of drugs called selective estrogen receptor modulators (SERMS)...preliminary results show raloxifene increases bone mineral density by 2 to 3 percent compared to a placebo and lowers cholesterol levels. Drawbacks associated with the drug include an increased risk of phlebitis, which is inflammation of the veins, especially deep vein thrombosis [conditions which precede one kind of stroke] and hot flashes."[37]

A study reported in *The New England Journal of Medicine* in February 1998 reported that Fosamex takers showed an average bone density increase of 3.5 percent at the spine and 1.9 percent at the hip, a fact that sounds impressive until compared with magnesium studies that show an increase of 8 percent. That's one reason the *Women's Health Letter* recommends trying magnesium supplementation first (see Part Two, Chapter 7). Another reason is that "Fosamex is so disruptive to the gastrointestinal system that it must be taken at least 30 minutes before the first food, beverage, or medication of the day...Then, you aren't supposed to lie down for at least 30 minutes and until after you've eaten. Fosamex actually works by interfering with the body's natural bone resorption process, and by doing so can lead to other serious health risks."[38] Biophosphonates such as Fosamex accumulate in the skeleton, where they remain for long periods of time. The long-term effects of such accumulation are unknown.

Another treatment in development involves gamma-Pyrones, which are inhibitors of parathyroid hormone. The focus of the latest ongoing research centers around Vitamin D analogues, in other words, chemicals that are similar in function to vitamin D, but different in structure. The hope is to create a patentable chemical that stimulates the cells that make bone bank deposits (in other words, an osteoblast stimulating agent or enhancer).[39]

Surgical Replacement of Bones

When bones finally wear down or break, some surgical procedures are used, for example, replacement of hip sockets, knees or shoulder joints, and sometimes even new ankles, elbows or finger joints. Currently about 125,000 Americans get new hips each year, and another 240,000 get their knees replaced.[40] Called arthroplasty, the joint is surgically reformed using a ceramic or metal ball with a plastic cup, sometimes cemented into place. This option yields positive results for some people, and it was for that reason Edith Crenshaw decided on it.

Edith was 75 when her bone health came crashing down. "I had more and more difficulty with motion of my arm, particularly putting it back to put on a coat. It got so bad I had trouble opening my purse, cooking, cutting bread, opening cans, holding the newspaper, and needlepoint had long since gone by the wayside." Her internist said it was a frozen shoulder and recommended some exercises that she did faithfully. They didn't help.

A new physician took a lot of tests and said the same thing. Then an orthopedist said she didn't have a frozen shoulder, she had erosion. "If you were younger and your livelihood depended on it," he said, "we'd do surgery, but it's a long climb up the mountain for a short ride, and we don't recommend it." After developing pain in her groin, she again saw an orthopedic surgeon. "He did the tests and said, 'we start the scale for hip surgery at 60 points and you're at 100, so you're a candidate for surgery.' I said, 'Hip surgery? What really bothers me is my shoulder!' So he checked that out. I was getting the pre-op lab work for the hip surgery when he came in and said I needed shoulder surgery. I went home steaming."

Her daughter picks up the story. "It was supposed to be a two-hour surgery. After four hours I called and they said not to worry, everything was fine, it would be another hour. After another hour and a half I called again and they said the same thing and it would be another hour. Finally I said, 'This is not acceptable; I'll go to the operating room and get an answer myself, or else you go in and get a direct answer.' So five minutes later they called and apologized."

It turned out that as her mother's surgeon had carefully completed his final micromovements to reattach the last muscle to her now rebuilt shoulder, her entire bone shattered, leaving the countless fragments in his gloved hand! Up until that moment, her osteoporosis had gone undiagnosed!

Now 76, Edith reports, "Once in a while I have really sharp pain in my hip, and limp, but it's very rare. I walk a lot better with a lot better mobility. I wouldn't go in for hip surgery now. I've been doing a lot of exercises, Tai Chi and water aerobics. I'm sure I have osteoporosis. My shoulder was evidence of it. It's only a question of how bad it is. I still have residual pain. On x-ray my hip looks like my shoulder, but I don't have the mobility restriction that I had with my shoulder. The surgeon recommended extra calcium, so I take that, and chondroitin sulfate and glucosamine."

In recommending she take extra calcium and the products to strengthen her connective tissue, Edith's doctor is addressing two points of the six-point plan. When I tested her during this interview using the method described in Part One, Chapter 4, I discovered she was also low in certain essential fatty acids, a third point of the plan.

Outcomes like these definitely reinforce the idea that it's better to get the body to repair its own bones whenever possible. But that's not the only reason. As orthopedic surgeon and author

Jason Theodosakis points out, "Even with the new joint, you don't have as much function as you did before...With surgery, there's always the risk of dying or becoming permanently disabled. And the surgery is painful, expensive, and not permanent—in ten years or so the replacement will begin to fail and the operation will probably have to be redone."[41]

Besides, that much bone bank capacity is also lost.

Treatments That Damage Bones

Some medical treatments for other conditions can set the stage for osteoporosis. In fact, some of the treatments now being offered for osteoporosis are damaging to bones! These include:

- Anticonvulsants (drugs used to treat epilepsy)
- Antibiotics
- Anticholinergics
- Cisplatinum (used in the treatment of cancer, it can cause excessive loss of magnesium)[42]
- Corticosteroids (used for conditions such as asthma or rheumatoid arthritis)
- Digoxin (used in heart conditions, it can stimulate magnesium loss)
- Diuretics (such as Lasix and thiazides, which increase blood calcium levels and can cause complications in conjunction with calcium and Vitamin D supplementation. Others can increase calcium requirements.[43] Some (hydrochlorothiazide, chlorathalidone, furosemide) promote magnesium deficiency.[44]
- Thyroid hormone replacement (too high a dose can stimulate bone loss)
- Sodium fluoride ("Women participating in a study at the Mayo Clinic in Rochester, Minnesota, were three times as likely to suffer from a fracture of the arm, leg, or hip if they

took sodium fluoride than if they took a placebo. Some of the participants also suffered from unusual lower leg pain, perhaps due to stress fractures."[45])
• Radiation exposure

In children, the most common cause of juvenile onset osteo-porosis is glucocorticoid therapy.

Surgery Can Affect Bones

Some surgeries, too, can have bone-crushing effects. Common surgeries that contribute to bone breakdown include removal of:

• gallbladder (cholecystectomy)
• ovaries (oophorectomy)
• stomach (subtotal gastrectomy)
• uterus (hysterectomy)
• prostate (prostatectomy)
• testes (orchiectomy)
• parathyroid
• thyroid

Noticeably absent from these medical options is any mention of nutritional approaches, and one must wonder why. One factor is that doctors are not taught about nutrition in medical school. A doctor friend of mine tells me that his entire nutritional education in medical school consisted of *one fifteen-minute segment of one lecture!* Alan Gaby, M.D., now President-elect of the American Holistic Medical Association, reports having been "told more than once in medical school to shut up about that mineral and vitamin research stuff, never mind that it's published in medical journals."[46]

And, this set of circumstances doesn't seem to be changing. Michael Janson, M.D., President-elect of the American College for Advancement in Medicine and President of the American Preventive Medical Association reports that most medical schools still do not teach nutrition. Adds Jean Barilla, M.S., "Through the early 1980s no medical school in the United States required a nutrition class. Today, several medical schools have added nutrition courses, but most do not address disease prevention and management."[47]

Why is this so? Funding for certain faculty positions, research projects and education is increasingly under the control of pharmaceutical industries whose primary interest is seeing to it that new doctors use their products. They put their money behind research that's likely to lead to development of patentable products. Nutritional products are not patentable because they are considered food, not medicine, so there is no profit in them for these companies. When companies find a food that works, they produce a chemical alteration or make a chemical imitation of it, which is patentable, and then send their product representatives around to the doctors' offices with glossy literature and free samples to "educate" the doctor. For particularly profitable products, doctors are offered continuing education seminars in Hawaii, or Barbados, or Palm Springs, where they will further their "education" about the patented product for a few hours a day.

This state of affairs is enforced through binding doctors to a legal standard of practice. That means that if they offer something different than the other doctors in their area, they can be sued and also have their license to practice taken away. So even if they are interested in nutrition and want to pursue it, they can be putting their careers and bank accounts on the line even to experiment a little. This is true even though medical literature abounds with information that nutritional approaches work. This state of affairs means most doctors keep their practices in line with the standard practice for treating osteoporosis. And the standard practice is limited to prescription pharmaceuticals and surgery. A suffering consumer who goes to a doctor expects to be given all the options known. But this is not the case: the options laid out to a patient by a physician will almost always be limited to the standard practice.

Does the source of funding actually affect the outcome of a study? Seventy articles, reviews and letters about calcium channel blockers were assessed for the author's position on the drug relative to the author's financial gain from drug manufacturers. Authors who supported the drugs had from a 37% to a 96% financial connection with drug companies.

"Interestingly, the people who researched these researchers do not believe that financial reumeration resulted in biased studies. We're not so sure about that (says the *Women's Health Letter*). If you conduct a large, expensive study for a company that's either lining your pockets or financially supporting a great deal of research for your educational institution, would you say the drug is of little or no value? If you did, do you think you'd be asked to be part of a future research project from this manufacturer?[48] Nonetheless, these same researchers often point a finger at nutritional information, saying it is inadequately researched, the fact that thousands of studies have been carried out notwithstanding.

The government agencies which could do something effective to change this situation actually work to maintain the status quo. Various departments which are supposedly independent are actually under the indirect control of the pharmaceutical giants. These corporations give large donations to the election coffers of officials who are "encouraged" to vote in specific ways or to appoint certain people to key positions in the governmental agencies that make relevant policies. Such appointed officials often have worked for the pharmaceutical giants prior to their government jobs.

Also, there is, says Dr. Julian Whitaker, M.D., "an incestuous relationship between the F.D.A. [Food and Drug Administration] and drug companies... Ambitious young ladder-climbers know that the best way to get high-paying jobs at the pharmaceutical firms is to put in their time working at the F.D.A."[49]

A treatment that becomes accepted as the standard of practice in the medical system is based on scientific investigation. This process, reports Dr. Dean Black, is to identify large samples of patients who all suffer the same condition; standardize treatments, so no variation can exist from patient to patient; hypothesize what will be found before finding it; hold confounding variables constant to keep them from contaminating the results; test for statistical significance; replicate the research, and submit it for peer review."[50]

The control of medical doctors by the pharmaceutical companies has been greatly aided by grants from the Rockefeller General Education Board and other foundations, which, since 1910, have sponsored so many grants to allopathic medicine that, in 1974, for example, nearly half of all medical school faculty received a portion of their income from foundation research grants, with over 16% being entirely funded in this way. Researcher Barbara Griggs concludes that this has hardly been disinterested philanthrophy, "since it eliminated all effective forms of alternative medicine for years, and promoted a monopoly medicine which is heavily drug-oriented."[51] This state of affairs has been further reinforced by the decision of JAMA, the Journal of the American Medical Association, to accept advertisements for patent medicines, which supplies more than half the A.M.A.'s revenue.[52]

So what is an afflicted person to do? Are there clinically effective options which are free of untoward effects and which support the body to create perfect bones? States Alan Gaby, M.D., "While collecting articles over the years, I came across many that suggested there is more to osteoporosis treatment than calcium, estrogen, and exercise..."[53] Indeed, to answer this question is to enter a different paradigm with different ways of thinking about bodily processes and healing.

It is exactly this shift Carol Gieg underwent when she changed jobs. Leaving the hospital where she was formerly employed, she moved farther north in California and began work as a mind-body therapist. As part of her new job, she began visiting healers in the area on behalf of her patients. This led her first to a chiropractor who showed her how to stretch and break up scar tissue which had formed in her muscles. He also referred her to a nutritional counselor. Using the method described in Part One, Chapter 4, the counselor recommended a clinical nutrition protocol (a plan including recommended supplements). Because her counselor was one of my teachers, she connected me with Carol to be interviewed for this book.

When I met with Carol, I found her well informed and articulate, and also very skeptical. After all she'd been through, I could see why she felt that way. But is such skepticism justified? Or is there hope that, even after two decades of searching, she could still find effective help? This was the dilemma facing her as she decided to be tested one more time to at least see what turned up. Using the same method described in Part One, Chapter 4 to make an assessment, we found evidence of weaknesses in all six areas of the Six-Point Plan for Perfect Bones!

This could certainly be greeted as bad news or good: bad that so many things were out of balance and in need of correcting, but good in that there are proven nutrition protocols to address and strengthen each area. Clearly not one to give up easily, Carol decided to proceed, taking the most important area first. We will follow her progress to see how she does.

Indeed, it is hard to believe that a new way of thinking might yield a different, effective plan of action. I understood this well, for I, too, was skeptical when I searched for what to do for my condition. I was up to date on current medical options, and I thought that if I knew those, I knew everything. Now, looking back, I am incredibly grateful that, even though I was unconvinced of the power of clinical nutrition, thinking that if it were any good I certainly would have heard about it, I proceeded with taking these protocols anyway.

If you might argue that these new ways of thinking about healing are unproven, you would be partially correct according to the research definitions used within the medical paradigm. Indeed, there are thousands and thousands of studies published in respected medical and scientific journals showing the benefits of clinical nutrition; yet these are largely ignored. If you wanted to use the idea that clinical nutrition has insufficient scientific studies as a justification not to consider clinical nutrition as an option, then you would have also to eliminate most of the treatments physicians use every day. Not only are many unproven, as we have seen, they can also be hazardous! If you want to wait until a treatment is "proven safe and effective" for osteoporosis, you will have to avoid all those listed above as well as the plan in this book!

However, your argument would be entirely incorrect within the paradigm of evidence-based medicine. In the evidence-based paradigm, proof of the effectiveness of a treatment is based on clinical results rather than laboratory experiments.

This different way of thinking is the subject of the next chapter, and its happy consequences for bones, the subject of the rest of this book.

ENDNOTES

1. Author's interview with Carol Gieg.
2. Jerry Green, J.D. "The Health Care Contract: A Model for Sharing Responsibility," from *The New Holistic Handbook*, 1985, as revised from *Somatics*, V.3, N.4 1982.
3. Alan Gaby, M.D. *Preventing and Reversing Osteoporosis, Every Woman's Essential Guide*, Prima Publishing, Rocklin, Ca., 1994, ix.
4. John Lee, M.D. "Osteoporosis Reversal, The Role of Progesterone" in *The International Clinical Nutrition Review*, Vol. 10, No. 3, July 1990, p. 384.
5. Arturo Corces, M.D., orthopedic surgeon, Cedars Medical Center. Summarized remarks at conferences on Osteoporosis and Related Bone Diseases, NRC, July 1997, sponsored by the National Osteoporosis Foundation and the National

Institutes of Health, Washington, D.C., June 1996 and July 1997.

6. http:// www.oxford.net/tishy/osteo.html

7. John Lee, M.D. *Natural Progesterone, The Multiple Roles of a Remarkable Hormone*, BLL Publishing, Sebastopol, Ca., 1993, p. 84.

8. J. C. Prior, "Progesterone as a Bone-Trophic Hormone" in *Endocrine Reviews*, Vol. 11, No. 2, May 1990, pp. 386–400.

9. Kerry Bodmer. "Editronate and Osteoporosis," *Women's Health Newsletter*, Vol. 7 No. 5, May 1998, p. 6.

10. Kerry Bodmer "Healthy Body, Healthy Bones," Ibid., July 1998, Vol. VI, No. 7, p. 1.

11. Kerry Bodmer. "Women's Health News, The Latest Healing Breakthroughs for Women, Summer 1999, p. 8.

12. Lee. *Natural Progesterone, The Multiple Roles of a Remarkable Hormone*, Ibid., p. 42.

13. Kerry Bodmer with Nan Kathryn Fuchs. *Stop Breast Cancer Before It Happens*. Soundview Publications, Inc. 1997, p. 16.

14. Kerry Bodmer, Ibid.

15. William Campbell Douglass, M.D. "Say Goodbye to Illness" in *Health Breakthroughs*, Fall 1997, p. 12.

16. American Pharmaceutical Association, via a grant from Sandoz Pharmaceuticals Corporation and the National Osteoporosis Foundation, January 1998.

17. John Robbins. *Reclaiming Our Health, Exploding the Medical Myth and Embracing the Source of True Healing*, H. J. Kramer, Tiburon, California, 1996, p. 151.

18. Eric Fidler. "Study: Osteoporosis drug lowers risk of breast cancer", for United Press International, *Ukiah Daily Journal*, Sept. 5, 1999, p. B–3.

19. Lee. *Natural Progesterone, The Multiple Roles of a Remarkable Hormone*, Ibid., p. 49.

20. Lee. "Osteoporosis Reversal The Role of Progesterone" in *The International Clinical Nutrition Review*, Ibid., p.389.

21. Lee. *Natural Progesterone, The Multiple Roles of a Remarkable Hormone*, Ibid., p. 47.

22. Wyeth-Ayerst Laboratories advertisement, *USA Weekend* magazine, Sept. 26–28, 1997, p. 11.
23. Gaby. Ibid., p. 139.
24. Bodmer. "Editronate and Osteoporosis", Ibid., Vol. 7, No. 5, May, 1998, p. 6.
25. Gaby. Ibid., p. 234.
26. Mary Ann Hellinghausen, Leigh Morgan, and Valeria J. Nelson for *NurseWeek*, June 23, 1997.
27. *Taber's Cyclopedic Medical Dictionary*, Eighth Edition, F. A. David Company, Philadelphia, 1960, pp. 0–23.
28. Bodmer. "Healthy Body, Healthy Bones", Ibid., July 1998, Vol. VI, No, 7, p. 1.
29. Gaby. Ibid., p. 233.
30. John R. Lee, M.D. with Virginia Hopkins. *What Your Doctor May Not Tell You about Menopause, The Breakthrough Book on Natural Progesterone.* Warner, New York, 1996, p. 169.
31. Mae Tinklenberg. *NurseWeek*, June 24, 1996, p. 21.
32. Alan Gaby, M.D. Ibid., p. 234.
33. Mae Tinklenberg. *NurseWeek*, June 24, 1997.
34. Lee. *Natural Progesterone, The Multiple Roles of a Remarkable Hormone*, Ibid., p. 68.
35. Alan Gaby, M.D. Ibid., p. 235.
36. Michael Dobbins, D.C., *Effective Nutrition Therapy*, a professional seminar, Berkeley, Ca., Feb. 28, 1998.
37. From Merck Pharmaceuticals advertisement for Fosamex; and Tinklenberg, Mae, M.S., R.N., "Healthwatch, Advances offer hope for treatment of osteoporosis," in *NurseWeek*, June 24, 1996, p. 24.
38. Bodmer. "Don't Let New Fosamex Study Fool You", Ibid., Vol. VII, No. 4, April 1998, p. 6.
39. Alan S. Levin, M.D., J.D., Author's Interview, May 1998.
40. Deborah Baurac. "Joint Exchange" in *Modern Maturity*, September–October 1997, p. 68.
41. Jason Theodosakis, M.D., M.S., M.P.H., Brenda Adderly, M.H.A. and Barry Fox, Ph.D. *The Arthritis Cure*, St. Martin's Press, New York, 1997, p. 3.

42. Gaby. Ibid., p. 40.
43. Balch and Balch, Ibid., p. 416.
44. Gaby, Ibid., p. 40.
45. Balch and Balch, Ibid., p. 416.
46. Jonathan Wright in Alan Gaby, M.D. Introduction to *Preventing and Reversing Osteoporosis, Every Woman's Essential Guide*, Prima Publishing, Rocklin, Ca., 1994, p. v.
47. Jean Barilla, M.S. "Rx for Health Care" in *The Physicians Newsletter, Health through Nutrition*, Jones Medican Industries, Inc. St. Louis Mo, Vol. 2 No. 1 April, 1997, p. 1.
48. Kerry Bodmer. "Update on Calcium Channel Blockers", Ibid., Vol. VII, No. 5, May, 1998 p. 5.
49. Douglass. "Say Goodbye to Illness," Ibid., Fall 1997, p. 12.
50. Dean Black. "Artful Science: Documenting the Chiropractic Experience, " Parker College, Occasional Paper, 1996, 1, as quoted in Clecak, Ph.D., "Giving Patients 'Reasonable Counsel': The Case of *Contact Reflex Analysis*, p. 1.
51. Barbara Griggs. *Green Pharmacy*, Healing Arts Press, Rochester, Vermont, 1997, p. 243.
52. Ibid., p. 238.
53. Gaby, Ibid., p. xiv.

CHAPTER FOUR

My Bones Are Not Your Bones: The Clinical Nutrition Approach

C an a new way of thinking lead not only to a new approach to the same difficulty, but also to different results? Instead of assuming, for example, that all bones are the same and will be healed with the same approach for all, where would the premise lead that all bones are different and need different approaches to heal? In other words, what if "my bones are not your bones"?

It was just this enigma I encountered as I became acquainted with the clinical nutrition paradigm through a muscle testing method called "Contact Reflex Analysis™", or "C.R.A.™" My local chiropractor had already figured out that my body needed calcium, and I had been taking an over-the-counter brand. But my back problems kept recurring; I'd suddenly have to put in a call because I was down on the floor and couldn't move. Because of chronic deep muscle tension that kept pulling my back out of alignment, he referred me to a health practitioner skilled in body work, Laura Samartino.

Soon after she began working on this muscle tension, she began training in C.R.A.™ and assessed me. I both dutifully and doubtfully began taking what was recommended for me. My progress seemed slow, I thought, but I reminded myself I was impatient after years of becoming increasingly decrepit, and I wanted results yesterday! When I heard that C.R.A.'s™ founder, Dick Versendaal, D.C., who had spent over 40 years developing this method, would be doing a seminar in my area, I decided to attend.

To say that my initial experience was dissonant would be an understatement. As a card-carrying, currently licensed, university educated member of the modern medical system, I had cut my teeth on Western medicine. I didn't understand that it had an underlying philosophy, nor did I begin to comprehend its implications until I heard the contrasting clinical nutrition approach. As Dr. Versendaal explained how C.R.A.™ worked and what it could do, my first responses were knee-jerk reactions right out of my medical model training. For a moment I was so stunned by what he was saying about the results of this method that I wondered why he hadn't been jailed for making false claims! Luckily the voice of reason also came forward and reminded me that it was just this method he was describing that had improved my health to the point where my body could tolerate a two and a half hour drive to the seminar and sitting all day in those uncomfortable straight-backed hotel ballroom chairs!

With considerable effort, I forced my former assumptions to sit in the back of the room while I opened my mind to hear him without prejudice. Listening, it finally dawned on me that the ramifications of this new approach were truly profound. If what he was saying were really true about the power of clinical nutrition to restore health, then the pharmacological and surgical approaches of the medical model were seriously restricted!

He used the analogy that "the body is like a computer and will compute anything you want to know if you know how to ask." This computer is made up of the brain, which operates not only like a memory bank, but also like an electrical generator, and thousands of miles of electrical wires or nerves. "These nerves connect every organ, gland and tissue of the body. They also connect with "fuses" or "breaker switches" called contact reflexes. By contacting these reflexes, using the body's muscular system as an indicator, we are able to monitor the function of the body systems."

This idea that the body has an electrical system seemed initially strange to me, but upon reflection, I realized Dr. Versendaal was saying the same thing I had been taught in physics and chemistry. All matter, the body included, is made up of molecules composed of atoms, electrons, protons and neutrons, every one of which is electrical. Electrical charge is a quantity of positive, negative or neutral energy present. In this case, it is present in a body tissue, but it is still expressed the same way. Chemically it is referred to as valence, and is caused by the motion of protons, neutrons and electrons. It manifests itself as attraction, repulsion or magnetic forces. It was this charged energy he was harnessing via an indicator muscle to test the state of the electrical charge of various systems.

And so I stayed the day as he tested these electrical reflexes in over a hundred people and outlined the corresponding clinical nutrition protocols. And, I also stayed the course with my own protocols. I continued seeing Laura and benefitted from her becoming a superb practitioner. It had taken twenty-five years to reduce my bones to their current porous state, we reasoned, so I'd have to give this method a chance to work, as indeed it did. As I began to experience greater and greater health improvements, I became more enthusiastic and also more curious. I began attending classes taught by Kim Sperry, C.N.C., a nutritional specialist of considerable knowledge. As it turned out, within a few years, not only had my bones recovered, but I was more active, vital, alive, agile and strong than I had been since my mid twenties! And, I had also undertaken clinical nutrition training so I could make it available to my clients.

A few years to restore complete health after twenty-five years of consistent bodily decline is not a bad bargain in my opinion. Still, why did it take so long? To answer that question is to delve further into how the body heals and how clinical nutrition works.

The Clinical Nutrition Paradigm

The clinical nutrition approach assumes that each of us is bio-chemically unique, so that even if two people with the same diagnosis are close relatives, each can require a unique healing strategy. Seven principles of clinical nutrition are significant for all bodily systems, including bone health:

1. the body wants to be healthy;
2. in addition to water and air, the body is made of only one thing (food);
3. in order to heal, the body uses food;
4. the body knows how to heal and will do so if supported with the right building blocks (in the form of food);
5. bodily processes can become so unbalanced that the concentrations of particular nutrients found in food are insufficient to restore balance and health;
6. foods can be concentrated to clinical potency and targeted to particular systems (including bones) so the body can heal itself; and
7. given enough time, the body will heal itself.

These principles are those that underlie holistic health approaches. They are expressions of the Empiric historical tradition, which is not a substitute for medical assessment or standard medical care. Rather, its aim is to balance the body and improve its vitality.

Historically, clinical nutrition has developed from roots that burrow deep into ancient healing traditions as diverse as the 3000-year-old Chinese acupuncture and the more modern (by comparison) school of empiricists or vitalists. Vitalists look at attitudes, behaviors, feelings, tensions, addictions, and pains as unique to each individual rather than applicable to all. They see these manifestations as disturbances in vitality, and, rather than seeking to eliminate symptoms, their approaches aim to improve that vitality. Stimulating growth or balance of the life force through nutrition is one such tool to improve vital energy.[1]

Muscle testing gradually became a way to assess the nutritional balance that contributes to improved vital energy. There are many systems of muscle testing. The greatly refined system of Contact Reflex Analysis was developed over the last 40 years by Dick Versendaal, D.C. Many of C.R.A.'s™ reflex points lie along acupuncture meridians, which are like "networks of microscopic nerves"[2] mapped thousands of years ago. Dr. Versendaal combined this knowledge with that of George Goodheart, D.C., on Applied Kinesiology™ (testing muscle strength) and with principles of reflexology and clinical nutrition, drawing from the work of Dr. Johnston and Royal Lee, D.D.S. He collaborated with a medical doctor, a dentist, a clinical nutritionist and a hematologist to research the nutritional protocols, and then assessed the results through independently conducted physical examinations, pre- and post-treatment blood chemistry analyses, urine studies and electrocardiograph comparisons.

The Clinical Nutritional Assessment Process

All practitioners rely on clinical experience to determine how to address their clients' needs. Some also use a variety of laboratory tests, which can include blood work, saliva, urine tests, and sometimes hair samples.

Michael Dobbins, D.C., teaches health professionals how to use a symptom survey form to assess their clients' need for nutritional balance. He is an internationally renowned lecturer in the field of nutrition therapy, a former college professor and instructor in the US Navy Nuclear Submarine Program. He describes how the symptom survey form works. "Every product Dr. Royal Lee made was designed to support one of the 12 body systems. These are assessed on the form through answers to 193 questions.

The one with all the check marks is the place to start [the healing process]."

To fill it out, he instructs people, "If it's what you're here for, put a 3. If I'd have seen you 6 months ago, and you'd have put it down, put a 2. If a year ago, put a 1. If you go, "hmmm", leave it blank. Most of it should be blank."[3] Then the practitioner scores it, either by hand or with new software programs (see Appendix: Sources). Some practitioners have people fill out the symptom survey form on the first visit and provide the report on the second. Some practitioners also offer a computerized printout of the results of the assessment (see Appendix: Sources).

C.R.A.™ practitioners often have clients fill out a symptom survey form to identify problem areas and have a baseline to evaluate outcomes. In addition, they use a method of muscle pulsing and resistance to assess what the body needs to heal itself.

But the last two methods, muscle pulsing and scoring, are at the heart of C.R.A.'s™ effectiveness. Scanning the electrical system of the body is profoundly informative, for the health professional can analyze some 75 different reflex points to assess what nutritional support is needed for every major organ, gland, system and structure of the body. The person being tested finds out which interventions, in the form of foods concentrated to clinical potency, are indicated to fuel the body so it can heal itself. Dr. Versendaal explains the technique:

> In a healthy body electricity flows to every area and feeds it the energy it needs to function. When you use C.R.A.™ to test the reflexes of each area, the testing arm, which is like a circuit breaker switch, will remain strong. There is no interruption of nerve energy. However, if one area of the body becomes unhealthy, it begins to draw excessive electricity in order to stay alive and functioning. This causes the body's electrical system to 'blow a breaker.' The testing arm will drop when the affected area is tested.[4]

This use of body electricity to assess the functional state of organs operates on the same principle as that which records the heart's electrical energy pattern with an electrocardiograph or EKG machine. But instead of using a machine, the practitioner contacts points on the skin surface, creating a circuit between it and an indicator muscle. The person being tested holds out an arm, and the practitioner presses down lightly while contacting each reflex in turn.

When any body part is injured or malfunctioning, its corresponding reflex-point shows increased electrical activity. With such an electrically "hot" reflex, the extra electricity is transferred through the practitioner and back to the test muscle, momentarily overpowering it so that the arm drops. "It's just like a wired fence," states Dr. Versendaal. "If you touch a wired fence and touch somebody else, they'll get the charge."

It is a method which can yield a veritable encyclopedia of information. It can also pick up tendencies toward disease long before they would show in laboratory tests. Nonetheless, states Michael Dobbins, D.C., former clinical professor, "Muscle testing is an art form and should be treated as such."[5]

A Perfect Ten

The method of assessing both the need for clinical nutrition protocols and their results is called "scoring". To score, the practitioner checks the electrical pulse of each organ to find out if the organ is properly charged, or is too high or too low. The focus of the nutritional protocols is to bring the level of the electrical charge back to normal, which, for most organs, is a ten.

Dr. Versendaal elaborates, "Back in 1912, D. D. Palmer, the original developer of chiropractic, wrote that too high or too low levels of energy in the body cause disease. Basically that's where we come from in C.R.A.™ If the energy in the body is too high or too low, it's the beginning of health disorders."

If the pulse of an organ or system is below or above a 10, Dr. Versendaal says "the person is a good candidate for C.R.A.™ If the assessment says the numbers are all 10, they're not a candidate for C.R.A.™ It's conceivable they could still have a health problem if everything's at a 10, but they usually do not."

He explains one way this concept relates to bones: "When bones have an electrical charge above a ten they may get spurs on them. A lot of people have these because the bone has too high an electrical charge. So they need to take Cataplex D (see Part Two, Chapter 7) from Standard Process. It reverses the electricity in bones and pulls that spur right back into the bone." (Note: If the number of the electrical charge on a bone is above a 10, it is important to rule out fracture.)

The Right Protocols

Once the assessment is completed, the practitioner designs a personalized clinical nutritional protocol. The recommended protocols are based on formulas developed by Dr. Royal Lee. Originally an inventor and electrical engineer holding over 100 patents, including some for guidance systems used by N.A.S.A., he became a dentist after designing dental equipment. Seeing a major increase in dental cavities, he concluded that "we are dying by the mouthful." To counteract this trend, he designed his first whole food concentrate, Catalyn (as the catalyst), that people could take three times a day. (For more about Catalyn see Part Two, Chapter 9.)

Westin Price, D.D.S., was another dentist who wondered the same thing. He studied the diets of cultures around the world, primitive groups who, if they died young, did so because of trauma, not because of degenerative diseases.[6] The ones that didn't have that happen to them lived to very old ages living on nature's diet.[7]

Clearly Dr. Lee was a genius and a pioneer in clinical nutrition, often referred to as the world's greatest nutritionist. In the 1920s, he founded the Standard Process company, which has continued to produce his formulas containing pure foods concentrated to clinical potency. The company grows its organic product ingredients on its own farms in rich, alluvial soil which has always been free of soil-depleting chemical fertilizers and herbicides and pesticides. They grow all the raw materials for their products. Their products are also free of coloration and coatings. These are some of the factors underlying the potency of Standard Process products.

It is a potency that is repeatedly demonstrated in clinical practice. For example, Mary Jane Mack, R.N., who practices C.R.A.™ in Seattle, Washington, and teaches it nationally, says, "I use only Standard Process products because I have predicable results. I know each month about where we're going to be and if something's not right. I know exactly what people need to do to get where they need to go for peak performance."

She adds, "I see people coming in who are on all these other products, and underlying they still have the same problem. I've been open to other products; I'm open for my clients' best interests, what's best for them, but I haven't found anything close to Standard Process. I see just about everything . . . every latest multilevel product, things other doctors and naturopaths have recommended. Some look like good products but just don't get the job done."[8]

Many products are made of synthetic vitamins, which are like a picture or model of the real thing: they are constructed similarly but have no life in them. Real food concentrates have life in them, and that life impulse is what can impart life to the body. The radiation of this life impulse can be seen in chromatographs, pictures of the quality of the color emitted by a substance as determined by its dominant wavelengths. As Judith DeCava, M.S., L.N.C, states, "It is simply a matter of chemistry versus biochemistry."[9]

The body simply does not know what to do with high dosages of these chemical isolates. It actually has to borrow the missing cofactors from its own nutritional stores to process such artificial vitamins, thus depleting the body further. And, as Dr. Versendaal points out, these counterfeit supplements can actually pollute the body, clog the elimination system, build up in the liver and create toxicity.

Many are "coal tar [or petroleum-based] reproductions of isolated chemical formulas of vitamin structures reproduced in a laboratory. They... also lack the synergistic elements normally present in whole foods... They often make you more deficient and out of balance and can create other problems because they do not contain all the cofactors [additional nutrients and enzymes] found in nature which made the vitamins work."[10] The synthetic vitamin products currently available, regardless of marketing, label or cost, are actually manufactured by a handful of chemical companies.

Michael Dobbins, D.C., states that "Dr. Lee concentrated food products and found out what created the greatest therapeutic change. Only later have some of the reasons why it works become apparent. One example is a vitamin which was named vitamin B4 when it was discovered there. However, it has never been discovered [meaning officially recognized] in the U.S." He adds, "Natural ones contain essential associated food factors in the form of enzymes and co-enzymes that are required for the full beneficial effects. Lee's products succeeded as much by their unknown factors and effects as by the ones that were known or are known. Many of the factors are still unknown."

Dr. Dobbins, who teaches clinical nutrition to health professionals, points out that synthetic vitamin B1 can irritate the peripheral nerve plates and create toxic symptoms. "The body does not have the enzymatic mechanism to ingest more than 5 milligrams of B1 per day; more than that results in female sterility by the 2nd generation. The symptoms of this overdose include fast pulse, irritability, tremor and weakness."[11]

But overdose is not the only problem. He adds, "The same template is produced whether by nature or by chemical synthesis, but it can bend with optical rotation (levo rotatory or dextro rotatory). In nature, these templates are found to be present about equally, about 50–50. The body takes the one it needs as long as trace minerals and other cofactors are present. But synthetic chemicals are all the same rotation. Therefore the body has to discard the half of the molecule it can't use. It's treated as a toxin by the body. The kidneys will always passively reabsorb something that's useful. But with synthetic vitamins, the body wants to use the half it needs, but is unable to extract the useful part because it's lacking cofactors. The dose is so high it burdens the kidneys and other body functions."

He continues, "The issue is not the molecule, it's the package. The person who is deficient can handle the food form, but they can't handle the massive dose of a synthetic. The body has to draw from its reserves everything it needs to handle this massive dose, and therefore becomes further depleted. It taxes the patient's body far too much. The body may not know the difference in a molecule of one nutritional factor, but it knows the rest is lacking. That's why there's a rebound effect. The end result is production of deficiency states that are worse than the ones they began with."[12]

A synthetic vitamin is a picture or model of the real thing; it is similarly constituted but has no life in it. The real food concentrate has life in it, and that life impulse can impart life to the body. The radiation of this life impulse has been scientifically demonstrated in chromatographs.[13]

Because many health care practitioners understand the significance of using real foods, they may recommend Standard Process products exclusively. This is because the body can indeed substitute chemical imitations of food in its structure. However, ingesting counterfeit and imitation food and chemicals can only attempt to compensate for their lack in their natural state. Informed practitioners point out that such substitutions are dangerous because they can actually weaken the body so that it easily falls prey to microbes when even a slight cell malfunction occurs.

The use of botanical nutrients rather than synthetically manufactured ones has been scientifically validated as far back as 1848 by Louis Pasteur, who discovered differences in their crystalline structure and molecular configuration. Organic molecules, it seems, are either left- or right-handed; thus their chemical makeup may be precisely identical but their crystalline structure different. The body not only knows whether it wants a right- or left-handed molecule, it also knows which one it is receiving and whether or not it fits. But pharmaceutical manufacturing processes cannot select for one or the other. Other, even more dramatic, differences have also been scientifically demonstrated; for example, chromatograms (measurements of color waves) show even greater disparities between synthetic and botanical nutrients.[14]

Bruce West, D.C., who produces the health newsletter *Health Alert*, also recommends Standard Process' concentrated food products: "I'm talking about products that truly change your body's chemistry, allowing it to heal. These are products that alter a heart graph, dramatically reverse pathological blood tests, alter organ and gland function that is proven on objective testing... The sad truth is that 95% or more of the things in your health food store and vitamin shop *cannot do this*. As such, if you are truly sick, they become a cruel hoax. There is just no way that I can recommend most of the products on the market today."[15]

He adds that "Manufacturers purport their synthetic products to be natural... In the meantime, companies like Standard Process Labs continue to pay attention to the soils in its organic fields, to yield crops high in phytochemicals (whole nutrients found in plants) and to render these crops into supplements in a miraculous, patented process that maintains the integrity of the health-rendering plant chemicals... in over 60 years, Standard Process Labs has developed and maintained its position as the *benchmark of excellence* in the entire industry *without ever advertising at all!*[16]

Standard Process' concentrated food products are also formulated with a different philosophy from most others. For example, their contents are designed to carry out a particular function rather than to contain a certain number of milligrams of an isolated nutrient. Their approach is "to give the patient the specific food factors which are lacking, along with the associated factors which make it work."[17] Thus labels may state that they contain far less of a nutrient in milligrams than manufactured vitamins. However, because that nutrient is accompanied by all the cofactors needed for the body to use it, fewer milligrams are required. And, of course, the converse is also true. Because manufactured vitamins are chemical imitations of food which lack the cofactors they need for proper absorption and utilization, greater milligram dosages are required to approach a beneficial effect.

One of the key differences in Standard Process' products is the presence in many products of substances called protomorphogens, or PMGs. Protomorphogens are the biological template for organs. They are complexes made up of nucleoprotein molecules, a phosphorus backbone, and a mineral substrate with as many as 60 to 90 trace minerals. They are also called 'growth factors' because without them, cells will fail to grow.

PMGs have an affinity for fibrin, which means they're attracted onto connective tissue. They provide the pattern by which the proteins will be built that become bone, or liver, or adrenal glands, for example. They comprise the sublying connective tissue of the gland.

PMGs are the smallest unit of the cell blueprint assembly. Without them, states Michael Dobbins, D.C., "the cell becomes senile and dies." He adds, "Some people have a failure at that level. They appear to have a genetic deficiency but it's really not. Their bodies are expressing a familial deficiency state that's been passed down for generations." Protomorphogens are especially powerful in such situations when the blueprint of an organ or system is functioning less than optimally. PMGs act like a guidance system that tells the nutrients to go to a particular organ to support it. Products containing them contain the letters "PMG" on the label.

Like fine wines, Standard Process' products reflect the conditions of air, soil and moisture under which their ingredients were grown; thus, the look of a product may vary from batch to batch. This fact reflects the living potency of the products. In other words, their products are formulated to give the body the living food it needs to heal.

Individually designed protocols are designed to be ingested daily over the length of a major healing cycle: a three-month period. Feeding the body the nutrients it needs during that three month cycle can result in a shift to regeneration from degeneration.

Evaluating Results

Most health care practitioners focus on *"functional outcomes"*, which means finding what works.[18] Dr. Bruce West refers to this approach as *"evidence-based medicine*: making observations to see what obviously improves the health of the patient... Evidence-based medicine involves trial and error... finding out what solves your particular problem... Keep in mind that what works for person A may fail for person B.[19]

In addition to clinical experience, practitioners using lab tests evaluate lab results to determine if their recommendations were effective. Practitioners using the Symptom Survey Form detect changes in groups of symptoms that relate to changes in the balance of particular organs, glands or bodily systems. For C.R.A.™

practitioners, says Dr. Versendaal, "a successful outcome is a 10 pulse on almost every organ and tissue of the body."

The use of functional outcomes and evidence-based medicine is good for the patient, but it can complicate the process of doing research. As Dr. Versendaal points out, "if you want statistics, you have to pick people you know you've treated for so many years, you have to work with hospitals to do lab tests. We don't have that kind of information. We don't have formal statistics."

"I've been in private practice 40 years," he adds, "and taken care of multiple thousands of people in a year. I've also had 7,000 phone calls in one year from people who want to come to my office. We couldn't take care of that many, but we got such positive results, people called and came from all over the world." Still, he says he "can't give numbers because people are going to say now get your records out and prove it. The only people that can produce numbers are full-time researchers, and often they're paid by big foundations . . . The bottom line is that it works."

Despite the challenges, the C.R.A.™ Research Foundation is currently tackling this project. Doctors from all over the United States are researching C.R.A.™ with clients and then sending in what happens to their clients' health using C.R.A.™ protocols. Research studies of C.R.A.™ and hundreds of positive peer reviews have continued to accumulate over the past 30 years. "At present, at least a dozen researchers/practitioners are conducting clinical studies of all aspects of this holistic healing art." C.R.A.™ is on its way to becoming "a vital part of mainstream health care . . ."[20]

Since formal research is just beginning, the number of people who have been helped to recover their bones using this approach can only be approximated as of this writing. One way of doing this would be to estimate that there are currently some 150,000 practitioners in the United States who use Standard Process products. If the rate of osteoporosis is one in six people, then one in six of these practitioners' clients would address nutritional imbalances that correlate with bone health. If each practitioner had only 60 clients, that would still be 10 clients each, or 1.5 million people.

Another way would involve estimating the number of practitioners Dr. Versendaal has trained. For the last several years, he has conducted three to four training seminars in the United States per month; each has been attended by 100–150 practitioners. Using the lower figures, 100 practitioners per training, times 3 trainings per month, or 300 practitioners per month, times 10 months is three thousand per year times 3 years is 9,000 practitioners. If each worked with only 50 clients during their whole time in practice, that would produce a guesstimate of 450,000 people.

I attempted an informal survey and discovered a range of responses. At one end of the spectrum are a variety of individual practitioners, many of whom work part time because they have young children. Each could be said to work with 5 to 10 such clients currently. At the other end of the spectrum is someone like Bruce West, D.C., in Monterey, California, who not only has maintained a longstanding, active, full-time practice, he also generates a monthly newsletter with subscribers across the United States. His approach to patients with suspected osteoporosis is also to balance their nutritional state. When asked how many patients with osteoporosis he had seen turn around in the process of improving their nutritional state, he replied, "Four thousand to five thousand."[21]

Elaborating further, he reported, "Most patients have osteoporosis. For most who suffer an osteoporotic hip fracture, I think their hips are broken before they even fall, and that's what makes them fall. The regular pressure and tension of the muscles and ligaments is enough to fracture a bone in someone who's osteoporotic. The osteoporosis is what's making them fall down in most of the cases."

Mary Jane Mack, R.N., has had a C.R.A.™ practice in Seattle, Washington, for many years. She also has taught C.R.A.™ for

Parker Chiropractic College as well as leading her own workshops all over the country. She says she has "helped lots of people prevent osteoporosis. That's what we do all the time." She estimates that over the course of her practice, she's helped maybe a hundred people who've been medically diagnosed. However, she reports, "I pick it up on a lot more, who are on the edge of getting it. I test for it myself using C.R.A.™ and follow the protocols."[22]

So, whether the number of people saved from this fate is 4,000 to 5,000, or 450,000, or 1.5 million, a lot of people have been relived from tremendous suffering. Nonetheless, from a scientific point of view, such information will continue to be considered merely anecdotal by the scientific paradigm of modern medicine until formal research is complete. And, vested interest being what it is, it's possible that positive results will be met with accusations that the studies were flawed.

Meanwhile, from a personal point of view, at the very least, these scientifically unaccounted for people are no doubt like I am, grateful every day for the powerful benefits of this healing method. They, too, must be very happy that they did not have to wait around while scientific debate took place and their health declined even further. Or perhaps they are too busy leading full and rewarding lives even to think about it.

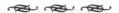

What, then, are the essential components of such an approach in the quest for Perfect Bones?

ENDNOTES

1. Jerry A. Green, J.D. "The Health Care Contract: A Model for Sharing Responsibility", Ibid.
2. Ron Shefi. "Contact Reflex Analysis" in C.R.A.™ Collector's Edition, an unpublished collection for professional education.

3. Michael Dobbins, D.C. "Effective Nutrition Therapy", a professional seminar, Berkeley, California, Feb. 27–28, 1999.
4. Peter Clecak, Ph.D., Ron Carsten, D.V.M., M.S., Paul Jasoviak, D.C., Mary Jane Mack, R.N., Steve Nelson, Pharm. D., Ph.D, Michael Robertson, M.D., J. Rodney Shelley, D.C., Donald Warren, D.D.S., FAHNP, "Alternative Healing Modes, A Look at Contact Reflex Analysis" in *Alternative Medicine Journal*, July/August 1994, pp. 10–13.
5. Dobbins, Ibid.
6. Westin Price, D.D.S. *Nutrition and Physical Degeneration*, Price Pottenger Nutritional Foundation, La Mesa, Ca., 1939.
7. Dobbins, Ibid.
8. Mary Jane Mack, R.N., Author's Interview, April 28, 1998.
9. Judith DeCava, M.S., L.N.C., *The Real Truth About Vitamins and Antioxidants*, Health Science Series #5, Brentwood Academic Press, Columbus, Georgia, 1996, p. 209 and pp. 216–221.
10. Fred Ulan, D.C., C.C.N., and Lester Bryman, D.C. "CRA New Client Orientation" in CRA *Collector's Edition*, 1996, pp. 2–3.
11. Dobbins, Ibid.
12. Dobbins, Ibid.
13. DeCava, Ibid.
14. Natural Vs. Synthetic (Is Natural Better?) in *The Nu Pro Therapist*, MPI NUPRO, Volume II, Number II.
15. Bruce West, D.C. *Health Alert*, Vol. 14/Issue 9, Sept. 1997, p. 1.
16. West, Ibid., 14/9 p. 1.
17. Training Session notes.
18. This principle is underscored in numerous writings about C.R.A.™, including the *C.R.A. Collector's Edition*.
19. West, Ibid., Vol. 14, Issue 5, pp. 3–4.
20. Clecak et al., Ibid., pp. 12, 13.
21. Bruce West, D.C., Author's Interview.
22. Mary Jane Mack, R.N., Author's Interview.

CHAPTER FIVE

The Bare Bones of Healing Bones: The Six-Point Plan

The working principle behind the Six-Point Plan for Perfect Bones is supporting nature's built-in process for keeping bones healthy. When bones first form in the embryonic stages of life, the necessary nutrients to make them are delivered via rich, maternal blood. Normal prenatal bone development depends on these nutritional factors being pumped in through the baby's umbilical cord. After birth, that job falls to our own blood supply. The quality of this blood, therefore, is central to bone health.

States Dr. Versendaal, "The number one cause of osteoporosis in my opinion is nutritional poverty: these people are living with poor blood. By the time most people reach 35–40 years of age, their bodies start running out of [nutrient-rich] blood. Up until that time they've been able to use the blood [legacy] their mother gave them, and that lasts them until they're 18 or 20. After that, they start living on cakes, cookies, candy bars and soda pop. The average American lives on junk food, and they're not going to get healthy blood from that."

He emphasizes, "Your body basically is made out of blood; that's what flows through everything. Each drop of blood has 250,000 red blood cells. You lose 3,000 to 10,000 red blood cells every second normally, and you replace 200,000 red blood cells every minute. All these cells have to be made by the bone marrow." Indeed, as he points out, bones and blood have a reciprocal relationship.

Healthy blood allows healthy bones to be made, and also, healthy bones contribute to the health of blood.

Bone marrow, then, is a crucial part of the bone bank; its rich stores are what the body draws on to maintain its health. Good nutrition "helps you build up your bank account so you can draw on it as you get older. You have to maintain your bone bank account so you can live on it and draw from it all the time." He emphasizes, "The only programs that work for osteoporosis are ones that feed the body blood builders . . . Blood builders contain ingredients that stimulate the production of blood. Vegetables, especially green ones that have a lot of iron in them, build blood . . . When you deal with somebody's blood, you're dealing not only with the bones, you're dealing with the whole body."

He underscores, "The good life is supposed to be the second half of life; that's when you want to lavish your body with rich nutrients. You don't think of your body using up your nutritional storehouse when you're young because you were born with it, but you've drawn on that bank by midlife. Then you need to make more deposits to draw on in the second half of life. Otherwise you'll pay a severe penalty in terms of health."

This way of thinking about bone health stands in contrast to the idea that bone health is a question of calcium intake only, or perhaps calcium and estrogen. Dr. Versendaal says he "can't conceive of bones simply being made out of calcium. My opinion is that since bones make blood, then they have all the resources in the matrix of the bone to make also bone, because bone makes blood, which is made out of vitamins and minerals, hormones, enzymes, hormone precursors, antibodies, vitamins and minerals. These materials are all in the right proportion to design our body, and they are made by the bones. Bones cannot be just calcium."

"Ironically," he adds, "the worst thing for older people is calcium. The reason is that calcium is electrically negative. It slows the heart down, and most older people have slow hearts. We're talking about the electrical charge, not pH, not valence. Most people have slow, weak, tired hearts. If you take calcium with blood builders like we do, such as e-Poise and calcium, you have a different electrical potential which is positive, not negative, and it can speed the heart up."

"When people who have a slow heart take calcium, it tends to slow their heart down, make the heart get weaker. They get tired, they cough more, they have more swollen extremities, they build up more water in their body. But if they take calcium lactate and iron or calcium lactate and a blood builder like e-Poise, there's a chain reaction as it [the water] pulls in to the positive electricity...Blood is electrically positive and when you build blood your body gradually retracts." This fact defines a relationship between osteoporosis and obesity.

The protocol listed in Part Three outlines the combination Dr. Versendaal recommends to build blood so that blood can build bone.

C.R.A.™ Assessment and Your Bones

C.R.A.™ practitioners assume, as does Dr. Versendaal, that "we have a tendency towards osteoporosis all our life if we're eating junk food. I think osteoporosis in many cases is nothing but bones that are overworked from trying to keep the blood alive when there are insufficient nutrients to keep the blood and the spleen healthy. The blood sucks the richness out of the bones...The bones have gone from being rich to being poor."

The medical criteria for diagnosing osteoporosis involve levels of checking bone density or urinary calcium output. C.R.A.™ assessment, Dr. Versendaal says, "gets into it further. The body is a whole and we feel you have to assess the entire body: the spleen, the blood, the stomach, the hormone glands, calcium levels, hemoglobin, and postural balance of the body to make sure there's not stress on the bones. We figure out how to balance the body so it doesn't stress out the bones and wear them out, so it has a perfect balance, a perfect flow."[1] He concludes, "Osteoporosis doesn't have just one cause, it has multiple causes ... You're taking care of a whole complex system of blood building contributed to by the bone marrow, the parathyroid gland, the uterus or prostate. All these organs are working together simultaneously to build bone."

Of all the 75 major reflexes tested in C.R.A.™, the one most closely related to bone is the heart reflex, Dr. Versendaal says, because the heart "gets its electricity from the bone marrow. The bone marrow in the sternum is [like] the battery. Your heart's right behind it. When the heart is tired and you sleep at night the heart draws off the sternal battery to stay alive. During the day when the heart is active, it [in turn] recharges the bone marrow."

Other reflexes, too, are significant for bone health. For example, someone with medically diagnosed osteoporosis or a subclinical case not yet diagnosed, Dr. Versendaal points out, might show weaknesses in other reflexes such as "blood quality, uterus, prostate, parathyroid gland, blood calcium, hemoglobin reflex, gall bladder, skeletal, gut reflex (digestion). There are plenty of people who get good food into their bodies but can't digest it."[2]

These reflexes show up in layers as C.R.A.™ testing reveals priorities for what to address first, second, and so forth. In fact, the body frequently does not even indicate the need to address bones directly until later in the process of healing. As Dr. Versendaal points out, "The body will always tell you whether or not something can be addressed without harm ... Nature knows best."

How might that process of discovering layers unfold? The story of my friend Sophia Tampinelli, a woman concerned not only about her bone health but about her overall health, will help answer that question.

Layers of Healing

To arrive at Sophia's house is to be welcomed with all the warmth of her Italian heritage. We first sat in her beautiful garden where the sounds of a splashing fountain and strains of opera floated on the evening breeze. Her kitty soon joined us, purring contentedly. Visiting her after returning from my first Versendaal seminar, I had enthusiastically reviewed what I had discovered, "You get tested to find out what your body is saying and then take the protocols to correct imbalances. Because the body shows what it needs in layers, you usually come back every three months, or once each season, to see what your body needs next, if anything. And each time you're getting your body in better health, and getting more and more finely tuned, constantly improving." As she had suffered recent and repeated bouts of ill health, she listened intently and decided to give it a try. Now I had returned to find out how things had gone.

First, we reviewed her history. An elementary school teacher, Sophia would turn 55 in another month, a ripe age for developing obvious osteoporosis. She reports that she is often 'bone tired'. No bone weakness has ever been medically diagnosed, yet she recounts many clues that her bones are not in the best of health: "feeling brittle, my back goes out easily, my left hip goes out, I have pain in my spine in between my shoulder blades. If I lean on my wrists too hard they hurt too." All this seemed to start, she says, around 15 years ago when she was 40 years old. To address it, she took up stretching exercises and saw a chiropractor a couple times a year. She also occasionally took some vitamins and minerals.

But this problem began, she thinks, in childhood. "I had poor teeth as a child. I relate that now to having malnourished bones. By age 20 I'd had all my teeth out. But that wasn't all. I started my period at age 8. At age 12 I had a D & C because I had a period where I hemorrhaged 40 days. I always had excessive periods. I had fibroid cysts on my ovaries too, so my hormones might not have been working right."

"I married at 18, and had five miscarriages when I was 18, 19, 20, 21 and 22. There were all kinds of theories about why—mostly it's God's will, or nobody knows, but nothing was ever found about why all this was happening. Besides, back then, doctors were gods and you didn't question." Still in her early twenties, she had a total hysterectomy. "After that I was on estrogen (Premarin) around ten years before I noticed scary warnings in the packages that said if you've taken it more than 6 months at a time there's an increased cancer risk. So I went off it, and have been on and off it for the last 20 years."

Then, six years ago she developed diverticulitis. "They took out a section of sigmoid colon and my gallbladder at the same time because I had a big stone that had bothered me for years. After surgery I gained 60–70 pounds and still haven't lost it all. I guess my digestion still wasn't working right."

We fell silent as the final rays of the setting sun cast its long shadows, then moved into her living room and settled on sofas. She continued. "Because I did massage about 25 years, I have an intense interest in health-related subjects. When I went to a conference on C.R.A.™, I got a lot of information. [At that time] I weighed 244 pounds. I was one of Dr. Versendaal's show-and-tell patients."

Layer One: But bones were not her first layer. "He said I had an enlarged heart and chemical poisoning. For that I took Parotid (a Standard Process product designed to support the body in removing chemical poisons. (See Part Two, Chapter 11.)

Layer Two: Then after my heart was stronger, he said to take the "sex hormone protocol". (This delay was because Dr. Versendaal was concerned her heart was too weak to handle the fluids she'd likely start to eliminate once she began the sex hormone support.) For this she began 1) natural ProGest cream and Standard Process' Utrophin, and 2) the core nutrition protocol (to improve her general nutritional status): 3 RNA, 3 Organic Iodine, 3 B6-Niacinamide and 3 For-Til B12. She reports, "I lost 24 pounds in a few months. I also felt my sense of well being return. I felt less brittle."

Layer Three: "He also found an indication that I needed nutrition to support gall bladder functioning, despite the fact that it had been surgically removed. This is because of a weakness in function rather than the organ itself." For this third layer, she took AF Betafood, which helps improve the quality of bile so essential for metabolizing the oils that carry calcium to the bones. These essential fatty acids are the precursors to every hormone in the body. "I'd always had trouble eliminating, but when I went on the AF Betafood, that changed. I felt clean and regular, with no toxic bowel and I was thinking better."

Layer Four: A fourth layer addressed parasites (for which she took Multizyme) and liver toxicity. "I feel we have been working on a causal chain, working backwards to get to deeper, more basic problems. I'm getting a better understanding of how it all works and what I need, especially the minerals. I'm from an Italian family, and I remember drinking wine as a child, but not milk. My father was from Italy, and he made wine."

Layer Five: Finally, after all the above protocols, her body indicated its readiness to heal her bones. She tested as needing two protocols: one for pituitary support, and one for bones.

Sophia's story demonstrates a basic principle of a holistic approach to health. As Jonathan Wright, M.D., of Washington's Tacoma Clinic, put it, "to take care of our bones, we must take care of our whole bodies and our overall health. What's good for the bones is good for the heart, the skin, the breasts, the stomach, and even crucial for future generations."[3]

Would the path of Sophia's protocols be right for someone else? Probably not. It was definitely different than my body indicated. Nor was it the same for Carol Gieg, whose search had taken her to eleven physicians. She discovered her own first layer when she went to Kim Sperry, C.N.C., the nutritional counselor from whom I learned C.R.A.™ Unlike Sophia's and my first layer,

Carol needed adrenal support initially. Her protocol included Cal Amo, a product to acidify her body and restore mineral balance, a calcium replacer, a whole food vitamin product called Catalyn, and flax seed oil. She had completed this phase when I interviewed her and assessed her next layer. Far from delaying her bone healing, concluding this first phase set the physical stage necessary for bone healing to occur.

Thus, C.R.A.™ has a double-edged health benefit. Using C.R.A.™ to improve the nutritional state of bones can improve the health of the entire body. And, addressing conditions not apparently related to bones indirectly improves the health of bones. Dr. Michael Dobbins, D.C., summarizes, "You provide nutritional support for a person who has a problem."[4] What, then, are the common denominators in such a healing program?

The Six-Point Plan for Perfect Bones

A truly effective program takes into account nutritional needs for all six points of the plan for perfect bones. To review, these are:

1. Healthy Connective Tissue
2. The Right Minerals and Their Helper Vitamins
3. Essential Fatty Acids
4. Hormones
5. Proper Absorption
6. A Clean Environment

The next section explores, each in its own chapter, each point of the Six-Point Plan for Perfect Bones. Each point has its own unique emphasis on building particular blood nutrients so that blood can build bone.

The purpose of this information is twofold. The first is so you can educate yourself about what you can do for your bone health. The second is so that when your health practitioner determines what emphasis your body needs, you'll be better able to stay the course and take the recommended protocols. You don't need to figure out which particular emphasis your body needs; your practitioner will do that. Your part is to understand what goes into building perfect bones. Then you are in a position to find a good practitioner, get a good evaluation, and take the recommended protocols. Your body will do the rest. A general protocol is provided in the last chapter.

ENDNOTES

1. Dick Versendaal, D.C., Author's Interview, January 24, 1998, San Jose, Ca.
2. Ibid.
3. Gaby, Ibid., p. vi.
4. Dobbins, Ibid.

Part Two

CHAPTER SIX

Building the Bank: Healthy Connective Tissue

Hard bone may seem to have little in common with supple ligaments, but actually, they are closely related. Connective tissue is the mother of bones. Without this healthy parental tissue, the daughter bones cannot form, or form properly. That's because bones are constructed on a mesh of fibers made of collagen (a connective tissue). In fact, connective tissue is referred to as "osteoid", which means 'bone-like'. Connective tissue is the protein matrix on which bones form. States John Lee, M.D, "Bones can be thought of as mineralized cartilage."[1]

Healthy bones are not brittle and weak; they are supple and strong. Connective tissue is what provides the suppleness. Therefore, to be healthy, bones need blood to carry nutrients rich in connective tissue builders.

Connective tissue is one of the four main tissues of the body. It binds together everything from the smallest cell to the largest organ. It's found everywhere in the body. It is what gives form to vascular tissues such as blood and lymph, its fibers making up the walls and holding the shape of all 75,000 miles of blood vessels, so blood can flow through them. In a body out of balance, these can become bony due to mineral deposits, a condition called hardening of the arteries, which contributes to dementia, strokes and heart attacks. A new technology, EBCT (electron beam computed tomography) can now produce computerized images of these arterial calcium deposits.

Connective tissues formed into strands and woven together form ligaments. These ligaments connect the ends of bones to other bones, to cartilage or to other structures where they either facilitate or limit motion. Connective tissue is also what supports visceral organs and keeps them in place so they don't all fall down on each other. Connective tissue also sustains the shape of intervertebral discs which keep spinal bones from rubbing together and crushing delicate nerves. Their fibrous network furnishes strength for skin, hair, nails, tendons.

Connective tissue also stores food. Michael Dobbins, D.C., points out that connective tissue holds substrates [the underlying substances acted on by enzymes] in reserve until cells need them and hormones stimulate their release."[2] Thus, connective tissue also plays a role in blood formation and some immune defense mechanisms.

Soft, pliant connective tissues turn into hard, strong bones through the efforts of bone cells. These cells use chlorophyll and green plant material to form proteins and trace minerals to produce an organic mesh. Once formed, this flexible fibrous net holds the various minerals that form bone in rigid, crystalline structures. The particular kind of protein mesh that makes up the bone bank's safe deposit box so it can retain mineral treasures is called collagen.

Collagen is the foundation for bone well-being. Without it, the body would merely be a mass of parts with nothing to hold it together. Given how important connective tissue is to every part of the body, keeping it healthy pays big dividends in the health of everything else. Indeed, when this mother-tissue disappears, the calcium and other bone bank mineral deposits that were bound to it go too. Without connective tissue, the mineral deposits that make up bone have nowhere to go.

Some connective tissue weaknesses make themselves known with a bang, others with a whimper. For me, it was a whimper of sorts, initially a matter of minor curiosity. There were occasional, small skin bruises in the winter, easily dismissed. There were fingernails breaking throughout the day. In summer hiking shorts and bathing suit weather, the bruises were bigger, so people often remarked, "Wow, what happened to you?" and point at a huge black and blue discoloration. "I don't know," I'd reply. But the bruises were so huge by now, if I'd banged into something that hard, I thought surely I'd remember hurting myself that badly.

Carrying the weight of the backpack with water and a few other supplies was now uncomfortable. I focused on building muscle strength, but felt like my muscles were working overtime. My back seemed to slip out of alignment too easily. By late fall I suffered an extruded disc.

Certainly the symptoms of someone else's connective tissue weakness might not show up the same way mine did. In fact, for many it begins as something they interpret as merely cosmetic. They look in the mirror and see the 'sag and bag' syndrome, or severe skin wrinkling. Uncomfortable about looking bad, some may even seek, not better nutrition, but plastic surgery. For tennis or racketball players, it may show up as 'tennis elbow'. Runners may develop knee pain. People who walk or stand may develop fallen arches in their feet. Someone else may have trouble keeping their bones aligned; they pick up a bag of groceries or a briefcase and pull their shoulder out. They throw a baseball and their elbow pops. They make a small jump and sprain their ankle.

When connective tissue is weak, muscles tighten, taking over the work ligaments were designed to do. But when muscles work overtime and connective tissue remains unrepaired, muscles, too, will eventually fatigue. Reaching this state, organs may drop from their proper place in the body, putting strain on themselves and other organs. Kidneys can drop, putting pressure on certain muscles and immobilizing others, causing the pelvis to destabilize and the sacroiliac joints to go out of alignment. The blood vessels in the lower G.I. tract may weaken, contributing to the development of hemorrhoids. The uterus or bladder also may drop, in severe cases leading to the recommendation of surgery to repair it. The ligament ring that holds the stomach in place may slacken, allowing some of the stomach and its acid to burn the esophagus, a problem often referred to as "acid reflux disease" or "hiatal hernia". When inguinal ligament rings loosen, they can allow portions of the intestine to enter them. Such an "inguinal hernia" is a dangerous condition, for the intestines can strangulate.

However the weakness makes itself evident, in terms of bone health, the relative condition of this connective tissue matrix is one reason why two people can have the same bone density while one suffers a fracture and the other does not. That's also why, at the level of connective tissue, the difference between the symptoms of osteoporosis and osteoarthritis tends to disappear and their relationship as disturbances in connective tissue can be seen. They are born of the same mother and, as members of the same family, express in different ways their mother's weakness.

For one person's connective tissue weakness may be due to a drug. For example, aspirin blocks the growth of new cartilage and accelerates joint deterioration. Another person's collagen deficiency may be connected to an injury such as a fall. Still another may have weak connective tissue due to exercise, or surgery. Being excessively over or under weight also plays a role. Some have weak tissue due to allergic reactions. For many, an alkaline pH has caused these tissues to erode. Some report that silicon breast implants started their connective tissue problems, leading to fibromyalgia, a debilitating condition characterized by extreme exhaustion, weakness and pain.

There are many other catalysts that can weaken connective tissue. One is the sun's ultraviolet rays, which, when they penetrate the skin's second layer, result in the skin wrinkling and aging. Two others are toxic substances produced by the body itself. Overstressed and weakened adrenal glands secrete a substance toxic to connective tissue, causing it to lose strength. Another is guanidine, a highly alkaline and toxic substance produced as a result of a toxic bowel.

However it starts, the decline of connective tissue health is like like the proverbial canary in a mine. It signals that bone health will be the next to deteriorate if something isn't done. States Dr. Versendaal, "You don't hurt bone as fast as you do connective tissue."[3] However the debility begins, doing something effective to reverse it is crucial to maintaining bone health.

Providing the raw materials this substance is made of helps keep it in the best possible shape.

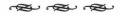

Connective tissue is built from certain essential building materials, primarily 1) protein, 2) silicon, 3) manganese, 4) Vitamin C, 5) Vitamin E and 6) Vitamin A.

Protein. Connective tissue mesh is made from proteins chained together. Proteins, in turn, are made up of chains of essential amino acids. Because these building blocks—essential amino acids—are heat labile (destroyed by heat), a sufficient quantity of raw foods is central to the health of this tissue.[4,5] Connective tissue weaknesses are much more likely to develop in people whose food sources are overcooked with little raw content. Among the best food sources for these amino acids are raw potatoes, jicama, raw mushrooms, the rinds of citrus fruits, and raw nuts, such as almonds or sunflower seeds.[6]

Silicon is an element found in more than one fourth of the earth's crust, usually in rocks and combined with other minerals. It is absolutely necessary to the health of connective tissue, yet when inhaled into the lungs, it can cause silicosis, a disease common to stonecutters. In the body, it is found in high concentrations at the calcification sites in growing bone. The collagen content of bones is diminished without enough silicon.[7] Apparently it strengthens the cross-linking of collagen strands.[8] Silicon is concentrated in silica in the form of silicon dioxide, and in horsetail and oat straw. It is also present in foods containing fiber. Since processed foods have much of their fiber content removed, people eating low-fiber diets may lack sufficient silica to keep their connective tissue strong.

Manganese helps prevent cardiovascular disease, maintains reproductive and nervous system health, aids in sugar metabolism and builds muscle. And, because it is an enzyme activator (helping enzymes to release their energy), it helps increase resistance to infection.

Manganese is the principle molecule around which collagen fibers organize themselves, which is why low levels are associated with abnormally formed cartilage and skeleton. It is the first material used to construct the place where bone mineral treasures will be deposited. Therefore manganese not only helps strengthen spinal discs and ligaments, it is crucial for healthy bones. "If the formation of mucopolysaccharides [used in forming connective tissue] is impaired by manganese deficiency, then the process of calcification (and consequently, bone formation, remodeling, and repair) will be impaired."[9]

Indeed, animals whose diets are deficient in manganese form defective bones. Professional basketball player Bill Walton discovered its role when he suffered repeated fractures which failed to heal properly without it. Manganese deficiencies are common in osteoporosis sufferers. Because manganese requires other cofactors, especially vitamin B12 as its helper, Standard Process' Manganese-B12 product contains both.

Good dietary sources of manganese are found in whole-grain cereals, nuts and legumes, especially rice bran and brown rice. As some products used to help heal spinal discs contain very large amounts of manganese, they should not be taken routinely, but only in acute situations until the body's need for them has been taken care of.

Vitamin C Complex. The whole complex that makes up Vitamin C acts as an antioxidant that helps protect the body from free radical damage. Many products on the market today are called 'vitamin C' but contain only ascorbic acid, a synthetic chemical imitation of one factor that makes up the natural complex. The complete food complex includes currently known components such as ascorbic acid and bioflavonoids, which include rutin, hesperidin, hesperitin, eriodictyol, quercetin, and quercetrin. These bioflavonoids are sometimes referred to as the Vitamin P, or vascular fragility factors in food. Their deficiency can contribute to bone abnormalities because they help keep the collagen fiber network tough. "One of the actions of vitamin C on bone is to promote the formation and crosslinking of some of the structural proteins found in bone."[10]

The role of the whole vitamin C Complex in bone health is profound. Sailors who spent long months at sea without benefit of fresh fruits found this out. A while after their gums began to bleed, their bones began to deteriorate badly, a condition called scurvy. Their sea captain finally brought aboard a huge stash of Vitamin C Complex-rich lemons (which the British call 'limes') to give his crew. That corrected their condition and gave British sailors a new nickname: limey.

It is important to remember, says Michael Dobbins, D.C., "A tablespoon of lemon juice a day cures scurvy, but massive amounts of ascorbic acid [which is missing all other parts of the complex] will not. The ascorbic acid made from synthetic chemicals also "seems to interact abnormally with iron and other chemicals in your body. The end result can be genetic damage or organ damage (as in the heart)."[11]

Vitamin C factors are found in blackberries, blueberries, cherries, raspberries and salmonberries.[12] Other excellent sources are in fresh citrus fruits, green tea, onions, cherries, plums and whole grains. Herbs with a high bioflavonoid content "include chervil, elderberries, hawthorn berry, horsetail, rose hips, and shepherd's purse.[13]

Remember that flavonoids or bioflavonoids do not take the place of vitamin C. Therefore if you're taking a product that has only vitamin C, or a product with only bioflavonoids, you're only getting part of what your connective tissue needs. Some authors suggest a 1:5 ratio of flavonoids to vitamin C. To be healthy, connective tissues need the whole Vitamin C complex, not simply ascorbic acid, which is the chemical name of one part of the complex. Many products labeled "vitamin C" contain only ascorbic acid, and therefore will not provide the connective tissue what it needs to grow strong.

Many ascorbic acid tablets are bound together with lactose (milk sugar), a significant problem for those with lactose intolerance. Unless the label specifically states, "No lactose" or "milk free" or "contains no dairy", it probably does contain lactose.

Because vitamin C complex is a water soluble vitamin, it is excreted rather than stored in the body, and must be consumed daily.

Vitamin E Complex. The contents of this complex are also called mixed tocopherols because they contain eight distinct molecules that "fall into two major groups: the tocopherols and the tocotrienols. Within each group, there are alpha, beta, gamma and delta forms.[14] It strengthens blood vessels, heart, lungs, nerves, pituitary gland, and skin. Because a deficiency is correlated with weak ligaments and flat feet, therefore it too must be considered as central to ligament health.[15]

The E Complex is fat soluble. Food sources include butter, dark green vegetables, eggs, fruits, nuts, organ meats, vegetable oils, and wheat germ. Wheat germ oil, available at health food stores, is rich in Vitamin E complex. Vitamin E becomes rancid easily. When it does so, it oxidizes to trans fatty acids, which cause more problems than they solve. That's why it's best to purchase it in small containers more often, or to use the Standard Process product.

Vitamin A Complex, a precursor to which is sold as Beta Carotene, speeds wound healing, supports connective tissue in skin, protects eyes against macular degeneration, and improves night vision. It is essential for development of healthy mucus membranes because of its role in the maintenance and repair of epithelial tissue. Without Vitamin A, the body cannot use protein, and therefore cannot build connective tissue. It was originally named 'retinol' "because of its influence on the development of the retina."[16]

Michael Dobbins, D.C., points out that "Vitamin A sold in the store is a beta carotene molecule that's a cheap, industrial waste product. Beta carotene is only one of many precursors which are later converted to retinol. He adds that many people, especially diabetics, can't convert beta carotene for use in the body.

Food sources include fish, fish liver oil, orange, green and yellow vegetables, milk products, liver, and orange and yellow fruits. Raw butter is an excellent source. The vitamin A in spinach is 10 times as potent as that from fish liver oil. Vitamin A is fat soluble, and therefore can be stored in fat cells and the liver. Therefore the body does not require it every day; however, because it is stored, it can build up in the body, resulting in hypervitaminosis A.

Other nutrients also play a role in creating healthy connective tissue, and therefore healthy bones. Among these is sulfur, which is a necessary stabilizing nutrient for "the connective tissue matrix of cartilage, tendons, and ligaments."[17] In so doing, sulfur is critical for maintaining the elasticity and flexibility of both connective tissue and fibrous cartilage. Sulfur is a component of all cells, but about half of the sulfur in the body is concentrated in the muscles, skin and bones. It is also prevalent in keratin, the tough protein necessary for keeping the hair, nails and skin healthy.[18] If you have arthritis, your sulfur levels may be too low. Sulfur has long been known to relieve joint pain and swelling, which is why sufferers find relief through frequenting hot sulfur springs. Foods especially rich in sulfur include meats, eggs and dairy products. Because sulfur has been depleted from our soils, supplementation may be necessary for some people.

The hormones estrogen, progesterone and testosterone also play key roles in the health of connective tissue. They direct processes that support the skin and mucous membranes all over the body. Therefore, maintaining proper levels of these hormones is central to collagen production and bone bank building. (See Part Two, Chapter 9.)[19]

Since the health of connective tissue underlies that of bone, what will strengthen it and keep it healthy?

If your connective tissue needs to be strengthened, your practitioner might find that a reflex called "master skeletal" tests weak, or that you have a spinal disc in need of healing. If so, you may have ligaments, muscles, tendons, or cartilage that need to be repaired. Luckily, you won't have to figure out all the major and minor nutrients that comprise it and then go buy them for yourself. There are good products already formulated for just such a purpose. Your practitioner will be able to test you to tell which combination will be the best protocol for you. (Note: Standard Process formulations are noted by (SP).)

Protocols

Ligaplex I (SP) provides the nutritional support to strengthen ligaments, and is often used for nutritional support in people with herniated discs, flat feet, chronic low back problems, poor ligament tone, ligament strain and in people whose backs won't hold alignment or adjustments. It contains a host of factors which support the ligaments, including manganese and vitamin E.

Acupuncturist and researcher Dan Newell, N.C., often recommends Ligaplex I (SP) "in acute situations for people who have herniated discs or who have high blood levels of calcium that precipitate manganese out of the muscles and ligaments. With herniated discs, they need the higher doses of manganese. It feeds the supporting structures around the discs."[20]

Ligaplex II (SP) is another nutritional supporter of liga-ments. It has less manganese concentration than Ligaplex I, and therefore is often used for people with ongoing, chronic muscle or tendon weakness that does not involve a herniated disc. Lee Vagt, D.C., advises people in acute situations to open the capsule and suck on it so it can be absorbed directly through the oral mucosa. He says that way it is absorbed directly into the nutrient bath (the extracellular fluid) of the body where it can be picked up (via passive diffusion) for the generation of new, healthy con-nective tissue. It contains the components in Ligaplex I in slightly different proportions, plus some additional factors used for people with degenerated ligaments.

Dr. Versendaal uses *Cal-Ma Plus* (SP) for repair of connec-tive tissue, especially spinal discs that are slipped, swollen or bruised. It contains calcium lactate, magnesium and a parathyroid tissue extract. (See also Part Two, Chapter 9.)

Many practitioners use the combination of 6 Ligaplex II and 9 Cal-Ma Plus for 12 weeks for connective tissue repair.

Allorganic Trace Minerals (SP). When low manganese lev-els are a problem, practitioners may recommend this product, which is high in manganese and other trace minerals, including iodine. For people who are sensitive to iodine, they may suggest Manganese-B12 (SP) instead, because it does not contain iodine. Both are high in manganese, which is "a muscle builder, bone hardener and ligament strengthener."[21] This product is useful when rehydrating the body is needed, especially to put moisture back in nerves when someone is jittery and can't sleep at night because the body is too acid.

Cyruta or Cyruta Plus (SP) contains ingredients from the green buckwheat plant. It is recommended if vitamin C Complex is the main nutritional need. It is rich in "P" factors (factors which, together, strengthen capillaries), including Vitamin C, inositol (one of the components of vitamin B complex) and bioflavonoids.

That's why it strengthens connective tissue. It's also used for people with high blood pressure and vascular fragility, which is why it sometimes is referred to as the "anti-stroke" vitamin complex. Since it contains the nutritional factors that strengthen blood vessels, it has the additional benefit of reducing migraines. It also supports the body to free itself of viruses (see Chapter 11). It contains many nutritional factors that support the capillaries for people who bruise easily or have "pink toothbrush", meaning their gums bleed easily.

Cataplex ACP (SP) supports both the production and maintenance of collagen. It contains the nutrients in Cyruta Plus along with the A and C vitamin complexes. In fact, the name "cataplex" means it contains the whole food: all the various factors needed by that particular nutrient to carry out its activity.[22] In addition to its use as connective tissue support for healthy bone, says Dan Newell, N.C., it provides the nutritional factors that "stop collagen overgrowth in such circumstances as adhesions from endometrial scarring, or after surgery." He has used it with success for people with deterioration of bone in the mouth: "ACP is used to get bioflavonoids in there in combination with Biost (SP, see Part Two, Chapter 7) which is the bone protomorphogen (the biological template composed of nucleoproteins)."[23]

If your connective tissue weakness is associated with night blindness, low resistance to infection, cystitis, and skin disorders, your practitioner may recommend Cataplex A (SP), which contains natural vitamin A esters.

Dr. Michael Dobbins points out that "it contains some of the best food sources for vitamin A complex...all the carotenoids... organic carrots, organic alfalfa, dried peavine juice (the single richest source of the full vitamin E complex), vitamin A esters from fish oils, nutritional yeast, rice bran extract and oat flour (the B complexes), vacuum dried adrenal, kidney, spleen, liver (for trace minerals and cofactors to sustain the health of the tissue, needed in micro amounts), mushroom powder (which contains a critical part of the vitamin C complex) and lecithin." He adds that rather than taking large doses of synthetic vitamin A, "small amounts of the right thing are far better than massive amounts of the wrong thing."

For-Til B12 (SP) may be recommended for low vitamin E level. It contains a special type of vitamin E in combination with tillandsia. It contains a high concentration of sex hormone factors (see also Chapter 9).

Wheat Germ Oil and *Wheat Germ Oil Fortified* (SP) are two cold processed products that contain whole vitamin E from wheat berries. See Chapter 8 for further information.

Protefood (SP) is recommended when connective tissue weakness relates to lack of the essential amino acids it needs, as when people eat overcooked food or show evidence of incomplete protein metabolism. They likely have other health problems such as viscous blood, decreased appetite, loss of muscular tone, cold extremities and fatigue.[24] One tablet a day is ample for people with extreme fatigue, while others may only require two a week, as it is highly concentrated.

One protocol for ligament strengthening for vegetarians is 3-6 spirulina; 3000 mg. vitamin C complex and 20 mg. of manganese per day.[25] These are available at your local health food store. In acute situations, for faster healing, he recommends holding the spirulina and manganese in the mouth to be absorbed directly into the blood stream from under the tongue.

Spirulina, or blue-green algae, is a "rich protein source (about 60% of dry weight) as well as a source of vitamin B complex, vitamin C and numerous trace minerals, especially iron, copper and zinc. It contains long-chain unsaturated fatty acids of the beneficial omega 3 type, such as EPA and DHA. A major cell component of spirulina is a sterol called chondrillasterol, which is a precursor of cortisone, a secretion of the adrenal gland. These sterols make up about 2% of the dry weight of some algae. Preliminary tests indicate that blue-green algae supports and enhances adrenal function and stimulates growth. In addition blue-green algae contains natural antibiotics and is an excellent source of healing chlorophyll."[26] As some brands of spirulina are not effective in strengthening connective tissue, be sure to have your practitioner test the product you want to use.

Lee Vagt, D.C., reports that some vegetarians have used sprouts in the place of spirulina. To be effective, he says, great quantities have to be chewed until they melt and turn to water in the mouth.[27] Another vegetarian alternative is a product from DC Labs called Discguard.

A different approach for vegetarians uses 6 Calcium Lactate (SP), 6 Linum B6 (SP) and 3 Organic Minerals (SP) a day.[28] The first two of these is covered in the next chapter; the third in Part Two, Chapter 8.

Sometimes weak ligaments are due to adrenal stress. See Chapter 9, Hormones for Bones, for protocols.

However it is strengthened, once this sturdy connective tissue mesh is in place, these flexible tissues are ready to receive the rich mineral deposits which will create strong, hard, solid bone, the second component of the Six-Point Plan.

ENDNOTES

1. John Lee. *Natural Progesterone, The Multiple Roles of a Remarkable Hormone,* Ibid, p. 55.
2. Michael Dobbins, D.C., Ibid.
3. D. A. Versendaal, Dick. D.C., Author's interview, Ibid.

4. Standard Process Training Session, p. 16.
5. Royal Lee, D.D.S., Ibid.
6. Lee Vagt, D.C., Author's Interview.
7. Alan Gaby., Ibid, p. 95.
8. Susan E. Brown, Ph.D. *Better Bones, Better Body*. Keats Publishing Company, New Canaan, Ct. 1996, p. 89.
9. Alan Gaby., Ibid, p. 31.
10. Alan Gaby, M.D. Ibid., p. 96.
11. Bruce West, Ibid., Vol. 15, No. 9, p. 8.
12. Lisa Lanucci. "Bone Power" in *Energy Times*, Jan. 1997, p. 18.
13. Balch and Balch. Ibid, p. 21.
14. Ibid, p.20.
15. Standard Process Training Session, Ibid, p. 13.
16. Ibid.
17. Michael Murray, N.D. "The true arthritis cure" in *The Arthritis Counselor*, Special Edition, 1997, p. 11.
18. "Sulfur an Ancient Nutrient Needed Now, More than Ever Before" in *American Council on Collaborative Medicine*, March 1998, Volume IV, Issue 3, p. 1.
19. Michael Colgan, Ph.D. *Hormonal Health, Nutritional and Hormonal Strategies for Emotional Well-being and Intellectual Longevity*, Apple Publishing, Vancouver, British Columbia, Canada, 1996, p. 117.
20. Dan Newell, N.C., Author's Interview.
21. Standard Process Clinical Reference Guide, p. 25.
22. This definition offered on audiocassette distributed by *Health America*.
23. Newell, Ibid.
24. Standard Process Training Session, Ibid, p. 17.
25. Lee Vagt, D.C., Ibid.
26. Raymond D. Schmidt. "A Treatment for Leprosy" in *Health Journal*, Price-Pottenger Nutrition Foundation, Vol. 21, No. 3, p. 1.
27. Vagt, Ibid.
28. D. A.Versendaal, D.C., and Dawn Versendaal Hoezee. *Contact Reflex Analysis and Designed Clinical Nutrition*, Holland, Mich., 1993.

CHAPTER SEVEN

Making Abundant Deposits:
Sun, Bones and Stones

Now that the connective tissue web for living bone is woven, the bone bank is ready to open for business and fill these supple collagen "safety deposit boxes" with mineral treasure. This magical transformation is one science calls "osteogenesis": forming and growing bone from connective tissue. Two types of nutrients take center stage in this process. The starring role goes to minerals, while the supportive cast is made up of vitamins.

To make bone deposits, minerals must enter the bone bank and then become anchored there, where they will form beautiful crystals (a form of hydroxyapatite). But minerals have many other places to go besides bones. In fact, minerals constantly move as part of a continuous cycle of regeneration. They travel from food to blood to bone to lymph to kidney and finally to urine, to be excreted. To get them to go into the bone bank and stay there, magnetic vitamins first attract minerals, then carry them into the bone bank and secure them. In this way, the entire bony skeleton repairs itself with fresh atoms of calcium, with the result that "adults typically replace their entire skeleton every seven to ten years" and "children replace their entire skeletons once every two years."[1]

One reason minerals continually shift is that they are called into service to keep the right acid/base balance, essentially in the neutral range—not too acid and not too basic. The right acid-base balance, or pH, takes top priority over strong bones, because bodily processes cannot function properly in an environment that's too acid or too alkaline. In its early stages, such a pH imbalance can cause cells to clump. Such lumps of cells can clog arteries and veins, setting the stage for heart attacks and strokes. A severe enough pH imbalance can cause death. To quickly rebalance pH, the body makes emergency withdrawals of alkaline minerals from its crystal bone bank deposits.

Many authors have linked a diet high in meat consumption with osteoporosis, assuming therefore that a high protein diet leaches calcium. This conclusion seemed even more correct after an Inuit Eskimo study in which scientists noticed a particular tribe had both high protein consumption and a higher than average rate of osteoporosis. However, as Michael Dobbins, D.C., points out, "The Eskimos had a higher than normal incidence of osteoporosis, but no causal link [between high protein and bone loss] was shown."[2] Perhaps what leaches bone is a high protein diet in the absence of dietary factors that rebalance pH within the normal range. Indeed, consuming a high acid-forming diet such as one composed largely of meat, fish and eggs without enough alkaline foods for rebalancing, could indeed leach calcium out of the bones and make them porous.

If the pH of bodily fluids is too alkaline, on the other hand, the body rebalances by rapidly drawing calcium out of bones and hiding it where it doesn't belong. The calcium thus taken out of circulation can form kidney stones and harden arteries. That's why it's unhealthy habitually to consume milk of magnesia or sodium bicarbonate; they create and aggravate an alkaline pH. Deposits of calcium into soft tissues can also be precipitated by a deficiency of phosphorus.[3] Most fruits and vegetables yield an alkaline ash when metabolized and thus don't deplete calcium stores. Whichever way the body is out of balance, it is likely to retain water and to become bloated or edematous.

You can test the pH of your own body by purchasing strips of testing paper in most pharmacies. Be sure to follow the directions on the package, and compare the results to the normal pH value for the bodily fluid you tested, i.e., urine or saliva. Remember, the lower the pH number, the higher the acidity.

Another reason minerals keep moving in and out of bone is that muscles require calcium to contract. The most important muscle of all is the heart. Keeping it beating is a top priority for life to continue, which is why the heart gets priority for calcium over any other muscle or bone. That's why the demineralization that makes bones unhealthy, if not corrected, can be followed by the loss of heart health. Fortunately, the converse is also true: improving bone health can precede improving heart health.

Luckily, the body gives much earlier clues than that of heart failure that the vitamins and minerals needed to crystalize bone are busy elsewhere, out of balance with each other or otherwise absent. Dr. Versendaal describes one such indicator, "A body with too many minerals and no vitamins to anchor them is a heavy body, big boned, thick skinned, thick hair. It's not necessarily sick, it just isn't loose or agile. However, a body that's out of minerals, probably because they're stored and can't be used, will lose hair on the head. That person needs vitamins to bring minerals out of storage so they can be used." Symptoms of such vitamin and mineral imbalances are not merely cosmetic, however; they are early signals that a process is underway that can lead first to porous bones, then to a malfunctioning heart and ultimately, to death.

When such a serious decline in bone health due to mineral and vitamin imbalance has already begun, reversing it can be a dramatic process. Such was definitely the case when my own body began to receive these nutrients in the right proportion. I had already been taking over-the-counter calcium supplements with minimal benefit. When I switched to Calcium Lactate (SP) (see below), I could feel my strength returning and my muscles relaxing by the hour. But that was my own story; I wanted to know someone else's. Renee Freeman, the caretaker of a woman with a similar experience, generously recounted one.

∽ ∽ ∽

"I take care of Berle Johns, who is 83, and her husband. They've been married 51 years. I do all their cooking and cleaning and taking them to the doctor. Anything that happens for them, I do. Berle had polio as a child and has a dwarfed foot, so she's always walked with a limp. But she was in a wheelchair when I started taking care of her because she'd broken her other ankle. Then in January she got a compression fracture in her back from doing nothing but bending over! If you can just bend over to pick something up and fracture your back, something's wrong!

"I took her to a nurse practitioner here in town, who ordered a complete body x-ray. Berle was in such pain during the test. The technician who took the x-ray said she'd never seen such thin bones. The doctor prescribed Vicodan (a pain killer) for her. Here was a woman who wouldn't even take an aspirin when she had her breast removed for cancer! Yet she was taking this Vicodan like candy. After 3 months the doctor said you've got to get off this.

"Late February I asked Kim Sperry, C.N.C. (a nutritional specialist and one of Pam's C.R.A.™ teachers) if she had anything that would build bones, and she did. But Berle didn't want to do anything, so I said to her, if you don't get up out of this bed and make an effort to turn this around I can't take care of you! I'm 60 years old myself. I said, Berle, you're going to have to pay for this medicine, Medicare won't pay for it. She has a doll collection, well over a hundred dolls. She was buying 1 doll every two months, so she quit buying dolls to pay for the medicine.

"So I got this natural stuff for her. She took Calcifood Wafers (SP), 6 a day (2 wafers 3 times a day). Then she also took Biost (SP), 3 a day for 6 months. I would say within two weeks' time the pain was gone and she wasn't taking any more pain pills at all. She was getting up on her own, I didn't have to lift her or help her in any way, where before I had to help her do everything. Before you know it, this woman was up cleaning out cupboards, doing the dishes.

"Her personality had changed too. She was much more open and she was dressed when I got there. She's got 150 cardboard boxes of stuff that's brand new and never even been used. I'd had to go through all the boxes because the cat would spray them. Now Berle's gone through the whole kitchen, cleaned out every cupboard. And, she's not yelling at her husband so much any more, where before it was constant. I was like a referee. She used to scream at him like you would not believe. One day I went down there and her husband had thrown a bread board at her and hit her at the chest. I said why did you do that and he said because she'd thrown a glass of water in his face! She's a changed person.

"Before she had this fracture she did nothing but sit on the couch and watch TV, not even combing her own hair or tending to her own needs. Now she's up at 6 A.M. brushing her teeth and combing her hair. She's moving around getting exercise too. The last time we went to town she didn't even use her walker! When you're around someone for several years and see how they are and then see the change, it's amazing. She marked down every time she took her bone stuff. She's got everything documented, she always wrote it down. She still has Vicodan pills but she doesn't take them.

"She's just taking a minimum dosage of this stuff now. She has not had any side effects. She's not taking any pain medications. She hasn't been to the doctor since January. It's unreal. She does hang on to furniture when she's walking because she has this terrible withered foot. Now I want to see if her nurse practitioner will do a full body x-ray to compare [the state of her bone health now].

"I have sent some of this stuff back to my husband's sister who's a nurse. Her condition is so bad she's on disability. She said she couldn't take it because it smells like something dead. I said, well, if you want to continue being on Vicodan and walking around like a zombie, you can just send them back and I'll give them to Berle!"

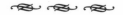

Magical Minerals

How could such a spectacular turnaround occur in such a short time? The two supplements Berle took were loaded with the minerals and vitamin helpers bones need. As Dr. Versendaal points out, such minerals make up a large percentage of the body. What exactly are these substances, that their deficiency could contribute to such a debility as Berle's, and their presence to such a dramatic recovery?

Technically speaking, minerals are a class of substances that occur in nature. They make up inorganic substances such as quartz, feldspar, and marble. They're also found in rocks, asphalt and coal. Minerals have a definite chemical composition and a distinct crystalline structure like those found in gemstones. Plants take these inorganic substances from the soil and convert them into organic forms, making them available for the crucial functions they perform in our bodies.

Eating a diet high in uncooked plant mineral sources is the best way to take in minerals. Raw plants contain both minerals and the vitamin helpers that are readily bioavailable, whereas cooking these green food sources, emphasized Dr. Royal Lee, makes them nutritionally relatively useless.

The list below contains some of the essential mineral gems that make up bone bank deposits, along with some other functions they perform. While learning about them, remember that it's not your job to figure out which ones you need and in what ratio. Nature has already done that for you, so that if you eat a balanced diet and avoid mineral leachers (see Part Two, Chapter 11), you'll easily keep a proper vitamin/mineral balance. And, if your body has levels low enough to require additional support, like Berle's apparently did, your practitioner can recommend supplements already balanced in the direction your body indicates it needs. What follows is merely to further highlight the significance of mineral balance.

Calcium. Calcium is a major mineral player in bone health, which is why it has received a lot of attention. In nature, calcium is found combined in limestone, coal, chalk, gypsum, etc. In bodies, 99% of it is combined in bones and teeth. "However, the remainder, a scant 1%, . . . circulates in the soft body tissues and fluids. Here it is used for normal bone and tooth development, blood clotting, enzymatic action and the regulation of fluid passage through the walls of tissues and cells."[4]

Calcium can quickly lower cholesterol; its administration has been demonstrated to decrease it by as much as 25% over time. Low blood calcium levels can result in low blood pressure, for the muscles that surround the arteries don't have enough calcium to contract. If calcium levels in tissues are too low, the skin can itch and even develop welts, especially when exposed to the sun. Getting sufficient calcium to the tissues can clear them up. It can also clear up viral canker sores inside the mouth. Viruses cannot enter the cells to replicate with sufficient calcium available.[5] Indeed, calcium is the "gas" that runs the immune system. When immune cells need to immobilize an invader (a process called phagocytosis), their cells send out little ladders and push; these are crystalline based and require calcium.[6]

Calcium administration can relieve back and neck spasms, menstrual cramps and even labor pains. In fact, administering calcium to one expectant mother I know played a role in her and her baby being saved from a C-Section she'd been told she'd require. Because her blood pressure was too high, doctors were afraid she'd have a stroke during the muscular efforts of labor. Her labor coach provided her with a calcium-rich protocol which she took every hour until her blood pressure came down, followed by a lower maintenance dose. Her blood pressure came down to normal, she delivered her baby girl normally, and the C-Section proved unnecessary. Calcium helps muscles do their work of contracting and relaxing, which is exactly what childbirth is all about. No doubt many women go into labor already in a calcium deficit, and then suffer great pain, even stalled labor when their muscles run out of calcium stores.

But even before childbirth, calcium plays a critical role in the health of pregnant mothers and their developing fetuses. Studies have shown that women who consume calcium during pregnancy can reduce the risk of pregnancy-induced hypertension and pre-eclampsia by as much as 70%.

However, that's not all calcium does. It helps coagulate blood, another critical factor in childbirth, but important even if you cut your skin or bump into something. Without sufficient calcium, a minor bump can turn into a major bruise. Calcium also helps nerves transmit their impulses. This may not sound terribly important until you think about what would happen if the nerve fibers in your heart lacked sufficient calcium to fire, or your heart muscle were too deficient in calcium to relax and contract. No doubt a great many heart arrhythmias and congestive heart failure problems begin and end with a lack of sufficient calcium.

These are a few of the reasons that, when body fluids lack sufficient calcium, they'll take it wherever they can get it. If sufficiently challenged, the body embezzles its own mineral treasure from teeth and bone bank deposits to keep going other systems more important to survival. This fact demonstrates the true nature of osteoporosis: it is a compensatory, life-saving adaptation designed to maintain life. Demineralizing bones is a way to keep the metabolic furnaces running and the heart beating. To the body's way of thinking, porous is better than dead.

Bruce West, D.C., summarized some of the common nuisance and moderately serious disease states related to the way the body uses calcium. His list includes "canker sores, herpes, shingles, kidney stones, sensitive gums and teeth, inability to handle heat, sunstroke, fevers, convulsions, certain types of heart arrhythmias, cramps, leg pains, and more."[7]

With calcium so essential to life, it is indeed shocking that "80% of women and 60% of men over 35 do not get adequate calcium in their diet."[8] Formerly, research to determine calcium need was carried out with college graduate students. New research conducted on senior citizens has demonstrated differing needs based on age, and the U.S.D.A. Human Nutrition Research Center on Aging recently increased recommended daily allowances for calcium.

But where to find it? Calcium-rich foods include dairy foods, asparagus, cauliflower, clams, beets, cabbage, carrots, celery, goat milk and cheese, onions, pumpkin seeds, turnip tops, kohlrabi, raspberry leaves, spinach, almonds, mustard greens, pinto beans, broccoli and tofu.[9] Additionally, because of public awareness about the need for calcium, some foods such as orange juice are being fortified with calcium.

Antacids have recently been touted as an excellent calcium source, but there are problems with this idea. For one, the calcium contained in antacids has a low bioavailability, meaning it's in a form the body has difficulty even accessing, let alone metabolizing. Two, proper calcium absorption requires an acid stomach environment, and antacids exist to absorb that acid (see also Part Two, Chapter 10).

Some researchers have estimated that perhaps only 10% of the calcium people ingest through diet or over-the-counter supplements is absorbable! In fact, a recent study examined whether or not increasing milk consumption protected against osteoporosis. The study population was vast: 645,221 person-years of follow up! It failed to show protective effects of dairy against osteoporosis.[10] Perhaps this is due to a problem nutritionist Royal Lee, D.D.S., pointed out as far back as 1955. He said that, as soon as it is drawn from the cow, milk is an unstable product because it is in contact with oxygen. He explained that once in contact with air, the milk sugar (lactose) reacts with certain amino acids in the milk protein, causing these proteins to progressively disappear. Those amino acids (particularly tryptophane and lysine) are the ones that are required to build tooth and bone. Pasteurization, he adds, completes this reaction so that it is totally incapable of rebuilding or maintaining bones and teeth.[11]

What about over-the-counter products? Again, the problem is bioavailability and ease of metabolism. "Minerals cannot be turned into tablets in their pure state [because they are chemically unstable]; they must be combined with some other substance or substances to make a stable compound."[12] This often renders them biounavailable.

The USDA-recommended dosages for daily calcium intake are significantly higher than the calcium-milligram dosages in the products Berle took, yet she recovered rapidly. The same was true for me. I took 6 Calcium Lactate (SP) a day, giving me a total of 250 mg. of calcium and 50 mg. of magnesium from that source. Yet my bones grew stronger. These experiences point to the power of whole food concentrates. All the calcium in Calcium Lactate, Calcifood and Biost is absorbable and assimilable. Therefore my body and Berle's could use everything in it. This was true for Berle despite the fact that, given her age (83), she probably suffered from low stomach acid production, which would reduce her ability to absorb supplements with a high milligram content of calcium.

Calcium intake is definitely important, but so is avoiding calcium loss once it's ingested. That means abstaining from substances that stimulate its loss. Such substances include alcohol, salt, sugar, caffeine, highly processed foods, phosphate-rich drinks such as colas, and a diet high in acid-forming foods, such as that containing excess animal protein.[13]

But is calcium always beneficial? In a word, no. Calcium that's ingested but not absorbed can be harmful. If you don't have enough acid in your stomach, your body will be unable to absorb it. Also, if you take calcium in the absence of magnesium, most of it will go straight through without benefit. And, that's if you're lucky. If your system is unable to eliminate it completely, the calcium you did not absorb can form stones which are stored in the gall bladder, kidneys or urinary bladder, causing excruciating pain. Addressing these symptoms medically involves uncomfortable tests and surgery to remove them.

When stored in the walls of arteries, it hardens them (arteriosclerosis); when deposited in the vibrating membrane in ears, it can make people hard of hearing. It can also calcify the heart valve. Clearly, the body makes no guarantees that it will deposit excess calcium where it can easily be removed by the surgeon's knife or otherwise. Calcium deposited in the wrong place can't always be surgically removed. A better option is to consume bioavailable forms in a high stomach acid environment.

Symptoms similar to those of metal toxicity can result from too great an intake of calcium or other minerals. According to Dr. Versendaal, these include: bloating, pitting edema, dizziness, chronic congestion, sinus trouble, high blood pressure, phantom pains, emphysema, coughing, asthma, ringing in the ears, A.D.D., cataracts, glaucoma, and Alzheimer's syndrome.[14] C.R.A.™ practitioners have protocols to support the body in eliminating such mineral overload.

As studies have shown, supplementation with calcium alone has had absolutely no impact on osteoporosis. Calcium cannot stand alone, without other minerals and the vitamins necessary for healthy bones. "[C]alcium is just one of many nutrients involved in the prevention and treatment of osteoporosis... bone tissue is complex, dynamic, and alive and, like other tissues in the body, has a wide range of nutritional needs."[15]

Magnesium. Magnesium is what makes fireworks burn and flashbulbs pop. Taken into the body, it is both an antacid and a laxative. In addition to being a component of bone, it also converts vitamin D to its active form, D3.[16] It is also necessary to help muscles relax, including those of the heart. It is sometimes used for nutritional support for patients with mitral valve prolapse, as people with this diagnosis often have low levels shown on lab examination.

On a daily basis, magnesium is essential for keeping bones healthy. In fact, some sources say the real problem in osteoporosis is lack of magnesium, not calcium. In fact, when several hundred women were given a reversed calcium-to-magnesium formula, their bone density increased by an average of 11%. That's a decade worth of bone loss recovered, assuming a loss of 1% a year in postmenopausal women.[17] You can ask your practitioner to check whether that's true for you.

Low magnesium levels not only are associated with porous bones, but, as studies in the U.S. and Europe have shown, also with developing arteriosclerosis and heart attacks, heart arrhythmias (irregular beats), high blood pressure and high cholesterol.[18] Indeed, magnesium plays a central role in keeping arteries strong. That's why health practitioners often recommend it for restoring strength to the coronary and other arteries.

Some research has shown that women's ability to absorb magnesium can drop so much that by age 70, we absorb only 2/3 of what we did at 30. One laboratory reports that most women over 40 test low for magnesium, a problem only intensified for those who eat poorly, drink alcohol or smoke, and take diuretics or anticholinergics. Stress, too, plays a central role in how much magnesium is available to the bones. When the adrenal glands put out adrenaline, that stimulates magnesium to be withdrawn from the bone bank.

As much as half the body's magnesium is found in bones. A "lack of magnesium is associated with abnormal calcium crystals in the bones, and normal levels of magnesium are associated with normal crystals."[19]

Its deficiency can also "cause various abnormalities of calcium metabolism, resulting in the formation of calcium deposits in places where calcium does not belong."[20] There are various opinions on what the proper calcium to magnesium ratio should be. Standard Process' Calcium Lactate product is based on a 5:1 ratio of calcium to magnesium.

Finding the proper calcium/magnesium balance is important for bone health, because too little magnesium can cause calcium to be excreted without being absorbed. Under this circumstance, the body extracts calcium from the bone bank for other needs, thus demineralizing them. Without magnesium, the body also cannot metabolize such essential nutrients as phosphorus, sodium, potassium, and vitamin C. Nor can it make crucial life-giving enzymes. On the other hand, too much magnesium can prevent any calcium consumed from being absorbed.

The right calcium/magnesium balance is important to heart health too. Calcium is necessary for the heart muscle to contract, whereas magnesium is required for relaxation in between beats.

Naturally, what each body requires to achieve the right balance is different, which is why nutritional protocols are individualized.

Dietary sources include whole grains, especially barley, and legumes, beans, and fresh vegetables such as chard, cress, corn, peas, parsnips, green cabbage, Brussels sprouts, endive, alfalfa and watercress.[21] Current USDA guidelines recommend a daily intake of 420 mg. for men and 320 mg. for women.

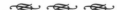

Phosphorus is as important to bone health as calcium, yet it has received much less attention. It's an element that is luminous in the dark. It's also flammable, which is why it's used to make matches. If the body lacks phosphorus, high tartar levels on the teeth and gums are likely to develop.

But phosphorus must exist in the right ratio to calcium. If there's too much calcium, the teeth can erode, a systemic cause of dental caries. States John Courtney, "Sometimes looking at animals gives you a clue about people. For example, take pigs fattened on grain. Grain is high in phosphorus. When pigs are young, usually about six months old, their teeth start to erode away because they are getting too much phosphorus and too little potassium and calcium."[22]

Some sources say the optimum ratio of phosphorus to calcium is 1:1. Other sources say the ratio needs to be 2.5 calcium to 1 phosphorus. After significant research, Standard Process arrived at a normal blood ratio of 4 parts phosphorus to ten parts calcium. That ratio keeps calcium in liquid form in the blood so it is available to be delivered to the bone bank.[23] When the body lacks sufficient phosphorus, it deposits calcium in tissues.[24]

Phosphorus and calcium are opposites that balance each other. Phosphorus holds calcium in solution in the body tissues during that phase of absorption in which bone bank mineral deposits are being delivered or withdrawn from bone. Thus phosphorus can actually prevent calcium from being absorbed if too much is ingested. That's one reason why drinking sodas is not healthy for bones: the phosphates in sodas compete with calcium. Likewise, too little phorsphorus prevents the body from being able to use calcium, no matter how high the calcium blood levels.

An example of how these two minerals affect the body was provided by John Courtney of Standard Process. He said that cattle raised in Wisconsin are big, easy-going and relaxed because they are eating grass high in the alkaline ash minerals, especially potassium and calcium. However, in Kentucky, where there are high phosphorus and low calcium levels in the soil, breeders raise not contented cattle but race horses. These animals are nervous and jumpy from eating grass high in phosphorus. They are loaded with energy and can't relax. Those same horses, when brought to Wisconsin, however, quiet down. The same is true of people, he says. If they're nervous and jumpy they need calcium. If they have no energy and are fatigued and worn-out all the time, they may need phosphorus.[25]

Iron. Iron promotes bone health, especially through its role in respiration: providing the oxygen necessary for the metabolic fires to burn brightly enough to transform food into muscle and bone. Iron is the mineral that carries oxygen in the hemoglobin molecule; without it, the body would suffocate for lack of oxygen. Iron is a mineral competitor with calcium, however, so when iron is needed for supplementation, it is best taken separately from calcium.

Trace Minerals

In addition to the major mineral players above, healthy bones need trace amounts of a variety of trace minerals. These include boron, zinc, copper, and strontium, among others. In a two-year clinical study, postmenopausal women who received calcium supplements in combination with zinc, copper and manganese demonstrated a gain in bone mineral density. However those taking calcium alone or a placebo showed increasingly greater losses. Perhaps this is because of the crucial role these minerals play in the hormone cascade that directs bone bank activity (see Part Two, Chapter 9).[26]

Boron. Boron may help the body retain and absorb its bone-building minerals. A recent study involved women age 48 to 83 taking 3 mg. of boron a day. "The boron reduced their bodies' loss of both calcium and magnesium...and the women taking boron actually saw a marked increase in their blood estrogen levels."[27] Their levels of testosterone also doubled (see Hormones for Bones).

Apparently boron reduces the loss of both calcium and magnesium as well as increasing estrogen levels. Studies have shown that when women have adequate boron levels, they can produce estradiol (one of the forms of estrogen) levels to equal those of women on estrogen supplementation.[28] Apparently boron plays a key role in the body being able to make both estrogen and testosterone.

Food sources containing boron include apples, raisins, grapes and pears, legumes, leafy green vegetables, nuts and grains.[29]

Zinc. Adequate zinc is essential to bone health because zinc helps bone cells (osteoblasts and osteoclasts) do their jobs. Without zinc, neither kind of cell could even form, let alone work! Zinc "further enhances the biochemical actions of vitamin D... and the synthesis of various proteins found in bone tissue. Zinc levels were found to be low in the serum and bone of elderly individuals with osteoporosis."[30]

Zinc is also essential in activating the digestive process (see Chapter 10). Zinc is a central ingredient in many enzymes that carry out thousands of different functions from cell growth to testosterone production. It also activates and boosts the body's ability to pick up nutrients in the gut and deliver them where the body needs them to be. Dr. Dick Versendaal, D.C., likens zinc to a substance that picks up nutritional hitchhikers. He emphasizes that the role zinc plays is so great that, when the body is deficient, other organs and systems deteriorate rapidly. These include the brain, pancreas, liver, eyes, prostate gland and nails. He points out that some 300 enzyme systems cannot proceed without zinc, including protein synthesis, vitamin D uptake, DNA synthesis, cell division, body growth, sugar metabolism, calcium metabolism, and skin, brain and stomach regulatory functions.[31]

Unfortunately for our health, zinc is easily replaced in the body by cadmium, a toxic heavy metal found in softened water, white flour, cigarette smoke and galvanized pipes in the presence of acidic water.[32]

Dietary sources include oysters, beets, broccoli, wheat germ and bran, milk, egg yolks, peas, beans, cress, liver, dandelion, lentils, seeds, spinach, fish, red lettuce, apples, cabbage and nuts.[33]

Copper. Copper "plays a role in the formation of connective tissue"[34] and helps to repair bone cells. So important is copper to bone health that horses grazing in the copper-deficient Florida Everglades become unusually susceptible to bone fractures, a condition corrected when copper is added to their diet.[35] Dietary sources include mushrooms, peas, leafy vegetables, seafood, red and black currants, whole grains, nuts, organ meats, eggs, poultry and legumes.[36]

Strontium. Strontium is an element whose compounds resemble calcium, which is why it can displace calcium in some processes. Like magnesium, it, too, is used in fireworks and flares. Unlike its harmful radioisotope, strontium 90, it is nontoxic and contributes to bodily health. According to Alan Gaby, M.D., "the human body contains about 320 mg of strontium, nearly all of which is in bone and connective tissue... Specifically, strontium is capable of replacing a small proportion of the calcium in hydroxyapatite crystals of calcified tissues, such as bones and teeth... [it] appears to impart additional strength to these tissues, making them more resistant to resorption... [and] appears to draw extra calcium into bones." He adds that its administration helps gradually eliminate any radioactive strontium.[37]

The trace minerals manganese and silicon have been covered in the previous chapter.

Vitamins: The Mineral Helpers

Vitamins activate every biochemical process. Without the help of certain vitamins, minerals cannot get into bones and strengthen them. Certain key vitamins bind minerals to each other and to the connective tissue mesh upon which bones form. Therefore they are essential to bone health. States Dr. Versendaal, "The majority of your blood is made out of minerals. The anchors to these minerals are vitamins." Two of the most important vitamins needed to deposit minerals into the bone bank are vitamin D and vitamin K.

Vitamin D. Vitamin D is essential for good health, and nowhere is a deficiency more expressed than in bones. A severe vitamin D deficiency leads to a disease called rickets in which bones cannot properly develop. Vitamin D provides the first phase of the courier service for minerals, carrying calcium and phosphorus from the intestine, or reabsorbing phosphorus in the kidney. Vitamin D takes these mineral treasures into the blood where they are ready for the next phase of their journey to the tissues or to the bone bank.

Vitamin D is made naturally by our skin. When we're exposed to the ultraviolet rays of the sun, cholesterol within the skin is converted to Vitamin D.[38] Glenn Miller, M.D., points out that "an area of skin six inches square exposed to the sun for about one hour every day provides the minimum daily requirement of Vitamin D.[39] Ten to 15 minutes of sun exposure per day is usually enough sunlight so the body can manufacture enough vitamin D. However, people who live in cold, cloudy climates where this is impossible may need to take Vitamin D during the winter months.

Some experts are concerned that people with darker skins who live in northern climates and people who take the anti-cancer message too far and use total sunblock creams may be falling short on their vitamin D. In the first case, skin pigmentation acts as a barrier; in the second, the sunblock does. A recent study concluded just that: sunscreens can lead to serious vitamin D deficiency. Researchers also discovered that the vitamin D content in milk is erratic. Many samples of milk advertised as containing vitamin D actually had none. Lack of vitamin D is associated with colon cancer, and is implicated in breast, ovarian and prostate cancer as well as in osteoporosis and hip fractures.[40] One large dose of 600,32 units of vitamin D "can cure convulsions and helps cure rickets."[41] Since the body makes vitamin D naturally from cholesterol, too-low levels of cholesterol can contribute to vitamin D deficiency.

Too much Vitamin D, called hypervitaminosis D, however, is harmful to health. High vitamin D levels can actually cause bone loss by leaking calcium from bones back into tissues. In a deficiency of its antagonists, which are contained in polyunsaturated fatty acids (see following chapter), Vitamin D takes calcium out of the bone bank and returns it to the blood, thus contributing to the development of osteoporosis. People taking a variety of over-the-counter supplements might actually develop this problem without knowing it, for Vitamin D is added to many products but not necessarily listed on the label. For this state of affairs, Vitamin F (see Part Two, Chapter 8) is needed, which is the natural antagonist to Vitamin D. With sufficient vitamin F present, the body will naturally balance production of vitamin D so as not to produce an overload.

The kidneys convert Vitamin D to the form needed for calcium absorption. Therefore, if the kidneys aren't working properly, they can spill excessive amounts of calcium. That means potential bone bank deposits are lost. (See Part Two, Chapter 10, proper absorption.)

Good dietary sources of Vitamin D include egg yolks, cod liver oil, salmon and cod livers, and butter fat. Bruce West, D.C., recommends raw butter as an excellent source of vitamin D for women who are prone to osteoporosis, skin problems, keratotic lesions, or even skin cancer. He reports the form of vitamin D in raw butter is in a form that is 100 times more effective than commercial vitamin D (viosterol).[42]

When vitamin D is actually present, fortified milk can be a source as well. Still, as studies completed as far back as the 1930s point out, natural vitamin D is "about 100 times more potent" than any synthetic version.[43]

Vitamin K. Vitamin K is often thought of as the clotting vitamin, but it also contributes to bone health by attracting calcium to the bone bank and binding it there in its crystal form. It is "essential for bone formation and repair; it is necessary for the synthesis of osteocalcin, the protein in bone tissue on which calcium crystallizes."[44] "Without adequate vitamin K, bones would lack structure and order and would, like chalk, be fragile and easily broken."[45] It's possible that postmenopausal women, the greatest risk group for onset of osteoporosis, have an increased need for vitamin K in the diet.

Vitamin K is found in fats, fishmeal, asparagus, blackstrap molasses, broccoli, Brussels sprouts, cabbage, cauliflower, dark green leafy vegetables (kale, turnip greens, spinach, watercress), egg yolks, liver, green peas, green beans, oatmeal, oats, rye, safflower oil, soybeans and whole wheat.[46] Good herbal sources include "alfalfa, green tea, kelp, nettle, oat straw, and shepherd's purse."[47]

Vitamin K is also synthesized by the benevolent bacteria that inhabit the intestines. As antibiotics kill these friendly bugs, it's important to bone health to replace them, both during and following a course of antibiotics. They are available in capsule or liquid form in health food stores, and can also be found in yogurts containing live culture. Labels often state "live lactobacillus or acidophilus culture".

Don't take products containing vitamin K if you are taking anticoagulants (coumadin, warfarin), however, as vitamin K interferes with the drug.

Vitamins C, A and E were covered in the previous chapter.

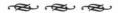

The challenge is where to get these vitamins and minerals. Although food sources are always best, if you think you can get enough of them to correct an imbalance by eating regular food in today's world, you might be sadly mistaken. For example, "Some researchers have said that as much as 90% of the calcium in pasteurized milk is not processed by the body."[48] Studies have linked the use of milk products "to a greater risk of coronary heart disease, other cardiovascular disease, cancer, diabetes, ulcerative colitis, lupus erythematosus, hypochromic microcytic anemia, kidney/bladder stones, female infertility, cataracts, gastrointestinal distress, colic, naso-pharyngeal allergic reactions, and muscle cramps during pregnancy. Consumers also must consider the possibility of contamination from agricultural chemicals, synthetic hormones or disease-causing organisms in some dairy products."[49]

Also, the soils in which these foods are grown are tremendously depleted of their vitamin and mineral content. In addition, many foods contain large amounts of pesticides or herbicides that can be toxic to bones (see Part Two, Chapter 11). Many foods also suffer from being overprocessed, which removes their remaining nutrients or renders them inert or unavailable.

That leads to the idea of taking over-the-counter mineral supplements. However, they are not problem-free either. One difficulty is that most are synthetic chemicals isolated from their cofactors, and therefore likely not to be assimilated. Another complication is deciding which chemical form to use; for example, calcium carbonate, or citrate, or what? Calcium carbonate is the form most widely purchased by consumers, but over-the-counter products are often difficult to absorb due to lack of proper formulation. This form of calcium is what produces the white filmy ring that appears after boiling hard water. This limestone (when put into products, called dolomite) is generally insoluble. That means it requires stomach hydrochloric acid to break it down, and thus uses this acid up very quickly. Dolomite has to undergo eleven biochemical changes to be absorbed, whereas the calcium lactate I took to heal my bones requires only two.[50]

To better understand this, suppose you were walking along one day and picked up a stone on the ground. You took it to a laboratory to see what it was composed of, and the report came back "1500 milligrams of calcium". If you then swallowed the stone, thinking you'd get your calcium dose for the day, you'd be sadly mistaken, for your body doesn't have a gizzard or some grinding machine to break down the stone and render the calcium available. Besides, if the calcium in the stone doesn't happen to be accompanied by its helpers, your body wouldn't be able to use much of it even if you could grind it down.

Many of the calcium products on the market are like that. A University of Maryland School of Pharmacy study in 1987 showed "that more than half of the eighty brands of calcium tablets tested . . . failed to meet the dissolution criteria."[51] This study was followed up by Consumers Union, which tested 7 brands and found 4 of the 7 failed to meet USP (the U.S. Pharmacopeia) standards. In many cases the pills were coated with shellac, rendering them insoluble by stomach acid: "The resulting product tended to act much like a slick pebble."[52]

They do not recommend dolomite or bone meal either, because "in the past, some samples have been contaminated with lead." Lead interferes with the hormone progesterone, which regulates the rate at which new bone is built. Oyster shells are high in calcium content, but our bodies are unable to access it. Chelated calcium is also ineffective. "Chelation purportedly improves absorption, but it actually does little more than raise the price."[53] They add that even if and when calcium supplements do meet USP standards, "you're better off getting your calcium from food."

Recently products containing microcrystalline hydroxyapatite, or MCHC, have become available. As extracts of whole bone, they provide the trace minerals and protein matrix necessary for the proper use of calcium. However, because most are heat processed, the protein matrix is destroyed, rendering them fairly useless, nutritionally speaking. However, if you plan to use such a product, make sure it has been analyzed for lead content, a common contaminant of bone meal products. Standard Process products are cold processed, leaving the protein matrix in place, and are free of such contamination.

The form of calcium the body can most easily use is calcium bicarbonate, which is given an electrical charge (ionized) through the action of enzyme systems. But calcium bicarbonate cannot be made into tablets "because as soon as you start drying the bicarbonate it changes to calcium carbonate."[54] The closest thing to it is calcium lactate. That's why so many practitioners stick to concentrated mineral/vitamin food products that are made from real foods and are bioactive and bioavailable. Then the body can readily, in one or two metabolic steps, deliver them to bone, where they are stored as dicalcium phosphate.[55]

Finally, before going on to nutritional protocols, a word about colloidal minerals. According to Dan Newell, N.C., "Colloidal means suspended. You could take rock and grind it and then suspend in within a fluid and it would be essentially the same as long as it did not pass through a semipermeable membrane when in solution. In sea kelp, the minerals are found in plants." Whatever their plant source, he adds, "The minerals have been organized and balanced by the plants themselves and were at one time in a colloidal state. Once they enter the body they are again in a colloidal state." Therefore the quality of a mineral product is not about whether or not the minerals in it are colloidal, i.e., suspended; it is about whether or not the minerals are bioactive, bioavailable, and balanced.

Protocols

To restore your own mineral and vitamin balance, your practitioner will choose from products that combine nutrients in the particular balance your body needs. These can include:

Calcifood (SP), one of the two supplements Berle took, contains in raw form the fiber and minerals for building bones and teeth, including calcium, phosphorus, protein and trace minerals. It is formulated in part from cold-processed raw bone meal which retains its biological enzymes. If the factors it contains are not being utilized fully, practitioners often add Biost.

Biost (SP), Berle's other supplement, supports bones, teeth and joints. It contains connective tissue protomorphogen, and manganese. It supplies the phosphatase enzyme the body uses to metabolize the raw materials that compose bony tissue.

Ostrophen PMG (SP) combines Calcium Lactate, Calcifood and Cal-Ma Plus to support the parathyroid. It "is lower in manganese and higher in raw bone meal, the little bit more that will often make the difference. It's a more complete package for bone or connective tissue repair, including osteoporosis."[56]

Bio-Dent (SP) is the protomorphogen extract (the DNA substrate) of bone used to rebuild bone, especially that around the teeth. It supports bone repair following mechanical removal of infection. Dr. Donald Warren, D.D.S., reports that use of 1-6 Bio-Dent tablets daily "results in a remineralization of incipient decays in approximately 50% of cases. At 10 per day, it has been shown to remineralize osteoporotic tempero-mandibular joints (TMJs) and the head of the femur."[57]

Calcium Lactate (SP) is so named because it is made from lactic acid, not dairy. It contains calcium and magnesium in a 5:1 ratio and in a form easily digested and utilized by the body. It is used to correct high phosphorus and low calcium imbalances, especially where dental caries and bone deterioration are occurring. It depresses high phosphorus levels. It helps improve all muscle functions, including those of the heart. It helps with fidgety, nervous energy, including in those who run high fevers. It may also be taken immediately at the onset of a cold, because infections easily take hold in a calcium-deficient environment. It is completely vegetarian. "It can be taken independent of food, as it will establish its own pH in the stomach."[58]

If your imbalance has to do with too little phosphorus and too high calcium, your body will be more alkaline. Alkalinity is involved in asthma, allergy, arthritis, bursitis, and infections as well as mineral deposit formation. To acidify it, practitioners may recommend products from grain food sources that leave an acid ash when metabolized. They act like the accelerator on a car and help the body speed up:

Calsol (SP) is a cereal source of calcium and phosphorus in a 5:3 ratio. It's a good source of phosphorus for vegetarians or lacto-vegetarians, and as such is a balanced product for long-term use by vegetarians. It's also good for hyperirritability, hyperperistalsis and muscular symptoms.[58]

Phosfood, (SP) may be recommended if you have a phosphorus deficiency and osteoarthritis, gall or kidney stones or tartar on the teeth. It also helps acidify the alkalinity of a high-calcium state when the body lacks phosphates.

Cal Amo (SP) is used to acidify the body when it is alkaline, and therefore sluggish, including sluggish digestion. It is used when the body lacks chlorides (rather than phosphates).

Organic Minerals (SP) are used in conditions of acidosis to alkalinize the blood, and with people whose thyroid (T4) pulse is too high (hyperthyroid). Organic Minerals are high in minerals that leave an alkaline ash, such as potassium and magnesium. They function like the brakes on a car, helping to slow things down, as when the heart races and muscles twitch due to lack of potassium. The minerals support the parasympathetic nervous system, including the vagus nerve, which results in a calming effect. This product is made in part from alfalfa, which is one of the deepest rooted plants and therefore contains many minerals from the different strata of soil the roots contact. Organic Minerals help the thyroid to rehydrate in situations where it has dehydrated, perhaps due to a viral infection.

Chezyn (SP) contains trace minerals of organically chelated zinc, copper and iron in a balanced ratio for when the body needs all three minerals, which may become evident in symptoms such as acne, poor soft tissue healing, blood sugar disturbances, poor immune responses and prostate disorders. It's also used to support the pancreas in people with pancreatitis.

Catalyn (SP) contains multiple vitamins, trace minerals and living enzymes. It is the original product developed by Dr. Royal Lee from substances that originate in the germ and seed portion of plants. Many practitioners feel that if someone only took Catalyn and nothing else, given enough time, they would eventually heal because it contains so many things the body needs, some of which are probably still unknown to science. Michael Dobbins, D.C., says "You can't overdo Catalyn because it's perfectly balanced." He recommends it to keep children's immune systems healthy in place of immunizations.[60] (Also see Chapter 9.)

He adds that "People are so grossly underfed now that 3 Catalyn a day won't do it. They often require 6 to 12 a day and up." He recommends chewing it for best results.

Because it provides enzymes and trace minerals that may be absent, Catalyn can provide the missing ingredients that make a nutritional protocol work.

Phytolyn (SP) contains clinical concentrations of kale and brussels sprouts. It is an excellent source of calcium in addition to having powerful anti-oxidant properties. Its calcium is bonded to the plant-based enzymes necessary for easy absorption and assimilation. Its minerals are delivered to bone along with the green plant substances they require to bind them to the collagen net.

Source of Life (by Nature's Plus) is a multiple vitamin product similar to Catalyn. It is completely vegetarian.

The following protocols are commonly recommended combinations, per day:

9 For-Til B12
6 Linum B6 for 3 months, then
6 For-Til B12,
1 Bio-Dent,
1 Biost,
2 Cal Amo,
1 Cal-Ma Plus,
2 Cataplex F Perles, and
3 Linum B6 per day always.

For vegetarians:[61]

6 Linum B6 for 3 months, then
2 Cal-Amo,
3 Linum B6,
3 Calcium Lactate,
400 units Vitamin D per day for maintenance.

Providing magical minerals and their vitamin helpers is only part of the equation in the quest for perfect bones. Once absorbed, they must be carried to the bone bank, a process covered in Chapter 8.

ENDNOTES

1. Dover, Ibid, p. 48.
2. Dobbins, Ibid.
3. Versendaal and Versendaal-Hoezee, Ibid.
4. "Calcium, Beneficial to Bones and More" in *Healthy Cell News*, Spring/Summer 1996, p. 17.
5. Standard Process Clinical Reference Guide, Ibid., p. 15.
6. Dobbins, Ibid.
7. West, Ibid., Vol. 15, Issue 5, p. 5.
8. Sharon Bortz, R.D., "Boning Up on Calcium", *Redwood Health Club Newsletter*, Sept. 1997, p. 1.
9. Mildred Jackson, N.D., and Terri Teague. *The Handbook of Alternatives to Chemical Medicine*. Oakland, Ca., 1975, p. 144.
10. Bob LeRoy, R.D. "Major Study Results Challenge Claims for Dairy" in *Vegetarian Voice*, Autumn, 1997, p. 19.
11. Royal Lee, D.D.S. Talk for the American Academy of Nutrition Society, Long Beach, Ca., April, 1955.
12. Balch and Balch, Ibid., p. 414.
13. Ibid, p. 415.
14. Versendaal and Versendaal-Hoezee, Ibid., p. 41.
15. Gaby, Ibid., p. 101.
16. Sutherland, Elizabeth. "A Natural Approach to Bone Health", Informational Letter to Health Professionals, 1998.
17. Kerry Bodmer. "Women's Health News, The Latest Healing Breakthroughs for Women", Summer 1999, p. 4, reporting on a study by gynecologist Dr. Guy Abraham.
18. As summarized in product information guide from Gero Vita Laboratories.
19. Gaby, Ibid., p. 42.
20. Ibid, p. 101.
21. Jackson and Teague, Ibid., p. 144.
22. Standard Process Clinical Reference Guide, Ibid, p. 30.
23. Standard Process Training Session, Ibid, p. 12.
24. D.A. Versendaal, D.C., *Contact Reflex Analysis™ Seminar*, San Jose, Ca., January 23, 1999.
25. Standard Process Clinical Reference Guide, Ibid., pp. 8–9.

26. Michael Colgan, Ph.D., Ibid., p. 229.
27. Douglass, Ibid. "Astonishing New Cure Reverses Osteo-porosis", Winter 1997, p. 12.
28. Douglass, Ibid., Winter 1997, p. 12.
29. Isadore Rosenfeld, M.D. *Dr. Rosenfeld's Guide to Alternative Medicine*, New York, Random House, 1996, p. 317.
30. Alan Gaby, Ibid., p. 82.
31. Versendaal, *Contact Reflex Analysis*™ *Seminar*, Ibid.
32. Nancy Appleton, Ph.D. *Healthy Bones, What You Should Know About Osteoporosis*, Avery, Garden City Park, New York, 1991.
33. Jackson, Ibid., p. 147.
34. Gaby, Ibid., p. 93.
35. Gaby, Ibid., p. 18.
36. Gaby, Ibid., p. 94. Also Jackson, Ibid., p. 145.
37. Gaby, Ibid., pp. 85–86.
38. Gaby, Ibid., p. 97.
39. Glenn Miller, M.D. "What are some benefits from exposure to sunlight?" *Ukiah Daily Journal*, Thursday, March 19, 1998.
40. Available: http://www.vvv.com./healthnews/dvitamin.html.
41. *Taber's Cyclopedic Medical Dictionary*, Ibid., p. V-230.
42. West, Ibid., Vol. 15, Number 9, pp. 1, 2.
43. G. Supplee, S. Ansbacher, R. Bender and G. Flinigan. *Journal of Biological Chemistry*, 141, 1:95–107, May 1936, pp. 95–107.
44. Balch and Balch, Ibid, p. 20.
45. Gaby, Ibid, pp. 22–23.
46. Balch and Balch, Ibid., p. 20; Brown, Ibid., p. 394; and *Taber's*, Ibid., p. v–24.
47. Balch and Balch, Ibid., p. 20.
48. Dobbins, Ibid.
49. LeRoy, Ibid, p. 18.
50. Clinical Reference Guide, Ibid., p. 29.
51. Balch and Balch, Ibid., p. 414.
52. *The New Medicine Show, Consumers Union's new practical guide to some everyday health products* by the editors of Consumer Reports Books. Mount Vernon New York, 1989, p. 204.

53. Ibid., p. 206.
54. Clinical Reference Guide, Ibid., p. 9.
55. Versendal, Author's Interview, Ibid.
56. Dobbins, Ibid.
57. Donald Warren, D.D.S., Author's Interview.
58. Versendaal, Author's Interview, Ibid.
59. Newell, Ibid., and Clinical Reference Guide, Ibid., p. 10.
60. Dobbins, Ibid.
61. Kim Sperry, N.C., Santa Rosa, California, designed all the vegetarian protocols listed at the end of each point of the Six-Point Plan.

CHAPTER EIGHT

Providing Courier Service:
Dry Bones and Essential Fatty Acids

How astonishing that an adorable, twelve-pound miniature daschund named Lulu could teach such powerful
lessons about the significance of the food group known
as "oils", or "essential fatty acids (E.F.A.'s)". Yet that was exactly
what happened.

She was living with a couple dozen others like her. The breeder
explained that Lulu, age 4, was going to deliver a litter of puppies
in a couple of weeks and six weeks later, when they were weaned,
we could have her. As it turned out, we didn't have to wait that
long, because Lulu gave birth prematurely. Of the two puppies,
one was born dead. The other had such a severe cleft palate that
it could not even be dropper fed, and it, too, soon succumbed. It
turned out Lulu had a history of not being able to sustain a pregnancy. The breeder was frustrated with the vet bill and no results,
and was ready to let her have another home.

But that was not the only clue that something was wrong.
Picking her up to bring her home, I remarked that her coat was
not shiny. The breeder responded by spraying something on Lulu's
hair to make it appear lustrous. As we got in the car to leave, the
breeder mentioned that an x-ray had shown that Lulu had a bony
spur in her spine, small and asymptomatic at the moment, but
likely to become a problem later.

Lulu seemed to adjust to her new life, but she still showed no
energy and no enthusiasm for anything: not a new bed, not food,

not toys, not treats, and not games! And, although my family spent considerable effort trying to get Lulu to wag her tail, she would not. In fact, she seemed to have no personality. I assumed she was grieving for her puppies and let it go. She would get aroused and alarmed, and bark from time to time, but she was never interested or curious. If I were to have seen that behavior in a human, I would have said she was clinically depressed. We poured on more love, gave her good food and went on with life, until several months later, when she began an alarming pattern.

Standing in the middle of the room, not moving or being touched, she would scream as if in excruciating pain. The vet gave her an ugly prognosis: Lulu had severe back problems which went with the breed. Luckily there was another vet nearby who specialized in back surgery. He would place rods in her back, and she'd be able to move around with a roller-skate-like contraption supporting her from midbody down, while she pulled herself with her front legs. Now she wasn't the only who felt depressed!

On an impulse, as I was leaving for an appointment with a health care practitioner who does nutritional work, I took Lulu along. This verdict was more hopeful. Nothing more was wrong with her than that she lacked certain oils. Add a teaspoon of olive oil a day to her diet and she'd slowly get better. The bony spur would gradually be withdrawn back into the spinal vertebrae. Give it three months.

And that's exactly what happened. Every day she became a little more mobile, a little more interested in life, more playful. By the third month she ran and jumped and wagged her tail. Her natural, affectionate, happy personality came into full flower. She'd run to the kitchen where her treats were stored, wag her tail ferociously, point her nose at the treat box and run back to the living room to arouse anyone who would listen. She even learned to roll over. She trotted happily along on six-mile hikes. She was back in the game of life, and she was playing to the fullest. And she stayed vigorous and full of zest until she finally died—of old age.

The Lipid Food Group

Such is the significance of oils in the diet that the lack of them can produce such profound symptoms, while their addition can effect such a powerful turnaround. Lulu's disintegration and recovery demonstrated some of the roles essential fatty acids play in health disturbances: hormonal insufficiencies, lackluster or unhealthy skin and hair, energy production disturbances, depression, and calcium absorption and delivery problems sufficient to create bony spurs and back problems.

I was to witness a human version of this in my practice when a therapist referred a woman of menopausal age whose major symptom was clinical depression but who did not want to take prescription anti-depressants. C.R.A.™ testing revealed she was severely deficient in certain essential fatty acids. (It is likely that the demand for EFAs, which are the precursors to hormones, is higher during the menopausal shift.) Unfortunately, that's also a time when many women are trying to force themselves to avoid fats in the interest of keeping their weight down and reducing heart disease risk. But actually heart disease is one outcome of lack of EFAs!

Whatever the reason, this particular woman was so depleted she had to take triple the usual amount (9 each per day instead of 3 each) of four products containing a variety of EFAs: Black Currant Seed Oil, Chlorophyll Complex, Linum B6 and Wheat Germ Oil (SP, see below for description). She pulled out of her depression in a few days and stayed out of it by maintaining her intake of these essential fatty acids.

How could oils pull someone out of a depression? For one thing, essential fatty acids are precursors for hormones. Essential fatty acids are the building blocks of fat in the same way that amino acids comprise protein. Besides providing building blocks for hormones, another reason EFAs can reverse depression for some may be that they provide fuel for the brain. According to Michael Dobbins, D.C., Ph.D., "The most efficient fuel for the brain is ketoacids, the breakdown products of fats."[1]

What are these powerful substances?

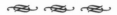

"Fats" or "oils" also are called "lipids", from the Greek word "lipos", which means fatlike substances. Membership in the lipid family is conferred on any nutrient which has the characteristic of being insoluble in water. It is a family whose relatives have some strange names. Some are called "true fats", which are esters of fatty acids and glycerol. Some are labeled "lipoids", such as phospholipids, cerebrosides, and waxes. Yet others are designated "sterols" such as cholesterol and ergosterol. Finally, others are referred to as "hydrocarbons" and include squalene and carotene.[2]

Some members of this family of essential fatty acids, also called vitamin F, make excellent dinner guests, while their cousins the saturated fats have received a questionable reputation in the scientific community. And one branch of the family, transfatty acids, is clearly toxic and dangerous, and best left uninvited.

The fatty acids to include are the polyunsaturated lipids the body cannot make, but requires for every living cell. The parents of this healthy family are linoleic acid (omega 6) and linolenic acid (omega 3). They help maintain normal growth (and the lack of it, as Lulu's puppies so painfully demonstrated). They also contribute to hormone production (including those which sustain pregnancy to full term), proper digestion and wound healing. Their presence improves the health of skin and hair. In fact, Dr. Versendaal has stated emphatically that there would be far less incidence (32,000 cases in 1997)[3] of malignant melanoma (skin cancer) if people were not so deficient in vitamin F, the essential fatty acids. EFAs also "reduce blood pressure, aid in the prevention of arthritis, lower cholesterol and triglyceride levels, and reduce the risk of blood clot formation."[4]

But that's not all. EFAs are also central to optimal brain and nerve function. "A deficiency of essential fatty acids can lead to an impaired ability to learn and recall information."[5] In part, that's because key brain nutrients must be carried to the brain in oil form in order to pass the protective blood -brain barrier. Also, the neurotransmitters the brain requires are made of EFAs. And, the layer of insulation around the nerves, the myelin sheath, is composed of fats (the ones named cholesterol, cerebrosides, phospholipids and certain fatty acids).[6] Without this protection, nerves cannot carry impulses from one place to another; instead, they misfire in a disorganized fashion.

This is a danger of cholesterol levels that are too low. Indeed, lower cholesterol levels are "associated with a greater risk of death from cancer and respiratory and digestive diseases."[7] Perhaps that is why the existence of some brain seizure disturbances has been linked either to a deficiency of EFAs or a disturbance in their metabolism. Children with hyperactivity and attention problems have "been found to be deficient in omega 3 relative to omega 6 fatty acids." Likewise, excessive anxiety and mood instability in adults may result from an imbalance between 'good' and 'bad' prostaglandins, a disequilibrium due in part to overconsumption of hydrogenated oils.[8]

EFAs—the welcome dinner guests (sometimes also called "cis form")—are made up of two groups: omega 3, or alpha-linolenic, and omega 6, or linoleic. Omega 3s are found in vegetable oils such as flax and chia seeds, walnut, pumpkin, and canola oil, as well as fish oil. Omega 6 EFAs are found in unsaturated vegetable oils such as soybean, primrose, sesame, grape seed, and borage. They are also contained in legumes, raw nuts and seeds.

Most food sources contain a mix of both types of essential fatty acids. But the one plant with the highest amount of EFAs, rich in omega 3, 6 and 9, is hemp. This plant is a cousin of the cannabis plant, but unlike marijuana contains no THC. It is more like hop or nettle, two other members of its family.[9] A relatively new source for Americans of these desirable EFAs is emu oil, either from California, or imported from Australia.

Whatever their source, EFAs support the body's defenses against high cholesterol, high blood pressure, rheumatoid arthritis and heart disease as well as helping decrease allergic responses and dissolve tumors. Omega 6s contain lignans, which are changed by intestinal bacteria into compounds highly protective against cancer, especially that of the breast. Additionally, lignans are also antibacterial, antifungal, and antiviral.

Michael Dobbins, D.C., points out that omega 6 fatty acids such as those found in red meats, organ meats and dairy fats, increase swelling (they produce arachidonic acid). However, when people consume no omega 6's, such as strict vegetarians, their liver gets a signal that more is needed and makes more. The result can be increased cholesterol levels.[10]

To address high cholesterol problems, some companies are now manufacturing epoprostenol, or prostacyclin, which are synthetically produced to attempt to "reverse vascular lesions". But the answer, emphasizes Dr. Dobbins, is to balance the ecosanoid system by proper eating. What might that mean?

Mary Jane Mack, R.N., recommends "olive, canola, butter. She emphasizes that people on low fat or no fat diets have the most health problems. "There's no lubrication in their bodies. They are open for osteoporosis because they lack the nutrients the body needs to function at a healthy state. Fat is necessary."[11] Dr. Dobbins concurs. "The higher the fat intake, the lower the incidence of breast cancer, according to the nurses' study, using 18,000 cases."[12]

The contribution of lipids to health actually begins with their supplying a continuous source of fuel the body can use or store through a process called thermogenesis, which increases oxygen taken in by cells. Any time extra energy is needed, the body can call on stores of these oils for energy. That's why competitive athletes add EFAs to their diet, and Alaskan sled dog mushers add flax seed oil, rich in EFAs, to their dogs' diets. By their very presence, these oils spare protein cell walls and cell nuclei from being broken down for energy production. Additionally, the presence of essential fatty acids makes possible the absorption of all the fat soluble vitamins: A, D, E, and K.

The right balance of EFAs, says Anne Louise Gittleman, M.S., "will allow you to lose weight effortlessly and painlessly without becoming preoccupied with dieting... Essential fat is the healthiest and easiest way to attain and maintain your normal weight.[13]

Essential fatty acids and bone health go hand in glove. EFAs can be thought of as the armored trucks that carry payloads of minerals on to their destination, the bone bank. "Vitamin F [these essential fatty acids] maintains a gut calcium level for the vitamin D to draw upon. Vitamin D can then pull the calcium out of the stomach and into the blood, and the vitamin F carries it from the blood to the tissues and bones."[14]

But EFAs can't do their job in certain circumstances, for example, when too many saturated fats are present. Their reputation has suffered a great deal lately, for rumor had it they were a chief cause of coronary artery disease. This idea is becoming increasingly more difficult to believe as evidence to the contrary is amassed. For example, the Eskimo diet was 80% fat for most of the year, most of it saturated.[15] How could they have even survived so long if saturated fats were so bad?

Still, the body does have to use up unsaturated fats to process saturated ones, so at the very least, saturated fats need to be balanced with sufficient unsaturated ones. Otherwise the oils that should be carrying calcium to bones are so busy getting rid of saturated fats that they never get down to one of the tasks they were intended to do, which is transporting new calcium stores to harden bones. An additional problem is that, due to modern farming methods, saturated fats can contain pesticide residues which interfere "with nerve function and oxidation processes in the human body."[16]

The outcasts of the family of oils, because they are toxic, are called transfatty acids. They result when hydrogen is forced into polyunsaturated oil molecules using high temperature and pressure, or when vegetable oils are constantly re-used, as in deep fried foods from fast food restaurants. Transfatty acids are found in margarine and any other product labeled "partially hydrogenated" or "hydrogenated".

Evidence is mounting that links these transfatty acids to a variety of health problems, including heart disease and cancer. The mass commercial refinement of oils has stripped EFAs from the diet and interfered with the formation of certain essential fatty acids (in particular, prostaglandins) that prevent tissue destruction and promote healing.[17] Michael Dobbins, D.C., points out that "transfats block the cascade of metabolic breakdown. They confuse the body; it uses the transfat instead of the good fat."

Some supplements, such as borage oil, evening primrose oil, and black currant seed oil, can bypass the transfat intake problem. However, EFA production can still be stopped by isolated fragments of nutrients like Vitamin E, aspirin, etc.[18]

The body uses essential fatty acids to make a variety of necessary substances. One of these is a steroid called cholesterol, which has recently suffered from a bad reputation also. But it is truly a required component of cell membranes, where it helps regulate the transfer of nutrients and waste products. Cholesterol is naturally produced by the liver in a process which is controlled by insulin levels. It is therefore the rise and fall of insulin levels associated with refined carbohydrates that seems to deserve the bad reputation currently pinned on saturated fats. Once manufactured, cholesterol is used as a fundamental building block for hormones and a coating for nerve fibers.

The body also uses EFAs to make over 200 kinds of prostaglandins, most of which are manufactured in the liver. They are hormonelike substances that serve as chemical messengers to help regulate the functions of cells. They control a variety of bodily processes, including arterial muscle tone, sodium excretion, blood platelet inflammatory responses and various immune functions.[19] Each needs to work in concert with the others. If one is out of balance, it can shut down the entire system.[20]

Certain fats promote inflammation because of the type of fat they contain. These inflammation-promoting fats exist in red meats, liver, dairy fats, shell fish and certain vegetable oils such as peanut, safflower, and corn oils. Other kinds of fats are inflammation-inhibiting, among them, olive, canola, evening primrose oil, borage, black currant seed oil, gooseberries, spirulina, flaxseed, english walnut, soybeans, wheat germ, chestnuts, spinach, beans. Because of their particular role in reducing inflammation, this second type of fat prostaglandin is helpful in any inflammatory condition, including arthritis.

The role of essential fatty acids in producing healthy bones cannot be underestimated. It's completely straightforward: no essential fatty acids, no healthy bones. EFAs carry the minerals and their vitamin helpers that bones need. And, EFAs are necessary ingredients to produce every hormone that directs bone bank activities. It is little wonder, then, that the incidence of osteoporosis is linked with insufficient dietary intake of essential fatty acids.

Porous bones are among the dangers of a low fat diet, especially when the small amount of fat eaten is saturated. A low fat diet exposes the body to the danger of having no carriers to convey new mineral deposits into the bone bank. Of course, there are numerous other associated problems, such as liver trouble and immune system breakdown. For women, too low a body fat mass is dangerous to bones. When body fat mass is reduced to around 15%, the menses may stop and bone loss (from low fat mass) begins. But too low a fat content in the diet can also damage the immune system, a fact Nathan Pritikin, M.D., found out. He lowered his body fat to 2 or 3% and his dietary fat intake to nearly zero in an attempt to avoid heart disease, only to die of leukemia. One wonders how his immune system could function with no essential fatty acids.

But too high an intake of dietary fat can also be problematic. It appears that high fat intake, when associated with high refined carbohydrates, contributes to a high incidence of heart disease. In terms of bone health, too high a fat intake creates a high level of acids in the bodily fluids. To neutralize these, the body draws calcium out of bones. Thus, long-term high fat intake equals greater likelihood of osteoporosis.

One attempt to deal with this problem has resulted in the manufacture of fake fats. One such is called olean, with the trademark name of Olestra. According to the Center for Science in the Public Interest, (CSPI) olean has been shown to cause diarrhea, loose stools, intestinal cramping and other gastrointestinal symptoms including fecal incontinence. Some people have even been hospitalized as a result of these symptoms. Additionally, fake fats rob the body of nutrients, in part by interfering with the absorption of carotenoids, a family of fat soluble nutrients that have been associated with lowering the risk of cardiovascular disease and cancer. Nonetheless, the Food and Drug Administration has approved its use.[21]

Some fatty metabolism problems are due not to too little or too great an intake, but rather to interference with their complete breakdown. Such disruption can occur in bulimia as a result of a pH shift. Interference with the complete breakdown of EFAs can also occur from taking anti-inflammatory substances such as aspirin, NSAIDS (non-steroidal anti-inflammatory drugs) EPA, DGLA and high doses of *synthetic* vitamin E. They all inhibit the breakdown of oils into their final metabolic product (specifically the PG 1, 2 and 3 series). Because these substances are incompletely metabolized, they make their own contribution to the inflammatory process, requiring more and more dependence on the anti-inflammatory substances whose complete metabolism they prevented in the first place. And, the body is deprived of the metabolic materials that would have been available and which it needs for other maintenance and rebuilding projects.

Still other fatty metabolism problems are associated with environmental circumstances. For example, in his travels to various cities in the United States, Dr. Versendaal has noticed that people who live near nuclear power plants are consistently deficient in essential fatty acids.[22] Apparently these oils are burned up rapidly in such surroundings. The symptoms such people show are the initial ones in an EFA deficiency. People become creaky, stiff, and freeze up, like the Tin Woodsman in the Wizard of Oz. They also build up sludge in the blood. Dr. Versendaal likens their condition to running a car 40,000 miles without an oil change. In the human body as well as in motor vehicles, oils lubricate all parts, help keep them moving, and keep the body clean by carrying refuse away. He adds that he finds lack of EFAs in men with prostate cancer, for which he recommends Linum B6 (see below).

Unfortunately, essential fatty acids are extremely volatile. "In their naturally occurring form, fats kink into a spiral, which means a great deal of exposure to the air; thus they have a high oxygenation rate and can easily become rancid."[23] When exposed to heat or air, these spiral-shaped fats partially decompose, in the process forming free radicals which are dangerous to cellular health.

Nutritionist Royal Lee, D.D.S., pointed out one such example. He said that one such source of essential fatty acids is lecithin. It contains essential fatty acids called phospholipids, which are hormone precursors that enable our glandular system to function. However, he emphasized, if it is refined, it actually promotes bone decalcification![24]

Therefore, how these oils are processed by the food industry has everything to do with their actual nutritional content once ingested. Unfortunately, most commercially prepared oils today are subject to a type of processing that negatively affects their nutrient value. "Expeller-pressed oils and hydraulic-pressed oils are first subjected to temperatures of 200 degrees F and up. The oils are then de-gummed, which removes chlorophyll, vitamin E, lecithin, and many minerals and trace elements. Then an alkaline wash separates out even more nutrients. Next, the oil is bleached and then deodorized by steam distillation at temperatures over 450 degrees F."[25] This oil then can be labeled "cold-pressed", a term that has no legal meaning.

However, the body knows the difference. No matter what amount of oils processed like this one consumes, the bottom line is the body begins to break down because it simply does not have the essential fatty acids it needs to carry out crucial functions.

Given how central essential fatty acids are to health, low levels of EFAs in the population should be considered a public health problem. "Breast milk and infant formula in this country have been found to have lower levels of the essential fatty acids omega 3 . . . as compared to European breast milk and formula. This fatty acid is necessary for proper brain and eye development in infants and mood regulation in adults."[26] And Donald Rudin, Ph.D., reports his research conclusion is that "Americans consume only 20% of the EFAs required for optimal health. Thus we crave food rich in fat and eat the wrong kind."

Indeed, EFA levels have been demonstrated to be significantly lower in people with heart disease as opposed to those who are healthy.[27]

Does the significance of essential fatty acids to bone health mean we should immediately increase our intake? No, not quite so fast: there is one essential precondition. The body has to be able to absorb and process them. That one prerequisite involves the gallbladder.

        ≈   ≈   ≈

The gallbladder is a small sac located just under the right rib cage, which is where its corresponding reflex will be "hot" if it's unwell. One of its functions is to concentrate the bile manufactured by the liver and release it in sufficient quantities at the proper digestive moment. It must function optimally for proper digestion of fats to take place. If its performance is poor or if the liver's bile production is faulty, oils will not be properly metabolized. Then they cannot do two of their essential jobs: carry calcium to bones, and rid the body of old minerals, metals and toxins.

The gallbladder's stores help break down and emulsify fat from food, and also help eliminate toxins. John Courtney from Standard Process provides an example: "If you create a lot of dust or if you work in a flour mill and breathe flour, it goes into your lungs where your blood picks it up and carries it over to the liver. The liver is like the oil filter in a car. It removes toxins from the blood and dumps them out of the body through the bile...which takes them to the intestines for elimination."

This process has been demonstrated by following the path of injected radioactive charcoal into the bloodstream with a Geiger counter. He adds, "If the bile gets thick like cream and does not flow smoothly, this indicates the person's fat metabolism is deficient. This is a symptom of gallbladder trouble. So we must thin the bile."[28]

Dr. Versendaal elaborates, "Your gallbladder's job is to retrieve from the liver all the minerals, including calcium, metals and toxins that are no longer useful to the body, in other words, they're electrically negative or dead. The body doesn't want them any more and sloughs them off, and the liver throws them into the gallbladder because it is loaded with bile which is very electrical. The bile pulls all those dead minerals out of the liver. Then the gallbladder has to get rid of them. If it doesn't, it makes stones out of the minerals it couldn't eliminate."[29]

Improving gallbladder health was the first layer of healing for me to get back my bones. It was also the first big problem Carol

Gieg began to correct after I saw her. Had we begun increasing our intake of essential fatty acids before correcting gallbladder functioning, we might have become sick indeed! Carol used 6 Betafood (SP, see below) a day for three weeks and then dropped to a maintenance dose of 2–3 per day thereafter, which is the standard amount.

That this protocol is effective can be seen in the reaction she had. A day or two after she began it, she reported an intensified muscle soreness. This was likely a result of her body now playing "catch up": finishing the job of metabolizing what it could not complete before. That is why she'd been instructed to take a week to work her way up to taking the 6 Betafood, so she wouldn't throw her body into a massive toxic reaction.

Actually, her response was good news, a sign that her bodily processes were getting back to work. Without this oil-metabolizing process working well, she would not be able to heal her bones. Dr. Versendaal explains how it works: "Betafood provides the nutritional support to get rid of waste, the old used up minerals and metals and calcium."[30]

Gallbladder functioning was also a problem for Sophia Tampinelli. As you may recall, her gallbladder had been surgically removed six years prior to her interview for this book. She'd had a big stone that had bothered her for years. However, after the surgery, she gained 60–70 pounds, her bone health continued to deteriorate, and the underlying problem of bile formation remained unresolved. Dr. Versendaal explains, "The job of your gallbladder is to retrieve waste metals and store bile. When you don't have a gallbladder, your liver is a backup, it has to do those jobs instead. Most livers can do it, some can't. When the liver can't do it, the person gets bloated, gas, belching, gets a huge belly from filling up with water, and can develop allergies, emphysema and psoriasis, even Crohn's [an intestinal inflammation] all from the liver backing up."

He describes the house of cards that can come tumbling down when the liver is backed up: "The unmetabolized oils turn to cholesterol. A lot of people have high cholesterol because their liver's backed up. The job of the liver is so awesome that any conceivable disease including osteoporosis can be brought on by the liver shutting down. The liver is a backup storehouse for the bone marrow to draw vitamins and minerals from, and the spleen is a backup for the liver. The spleen's job is to take the damaged blood cells and make them new again. When the liver can't manage any more, the spleen takes over. But if the spleen, too, gets overwhelmed and shuts down, the body not only robs the bone marrow, it also has to work harder to repair the blood cells the spleen's not repairing. The better the spleen works, the better the bone marrow. That's how the body balances itself."[31]

Crystal M. had the unfortunate distinction of finding out the truth of Dr. Versendaal's words and the gallbladder's connection to bone health: "My gallbladder has probably not been working optimally all my life," she said. "I have been plagued with constipation since birth. As a young woman in my late twenties, digestive and other problems prompted a chiropractor to recommend a gallbladder cleanse. The regimen involved fasting, taking powerful laxatives, and ingesting a mixture of olive oil and citrus juice. It worked. I eliminated more than a cup of stones as large as marbles. It was painful, but not horrible. I tried it again several other times but had to stop."

However, the problem was still not solved. She continued to have light stools, a classic sign of gallbladder problems. She continues, "Along the way I learned to reduce or eliminate fatty foods due to the pain and problems they caused [which no doubt contributed significantly to her lack of essential fatty acids]. In the meantime, by age 45 I developed severe osteoporosis. It was explained to me by my C.R.A.™ consultant that essential fatty acids are needed to carry calcium to the bones. Lo and behold, gallbladder emerged as needing support during a C.R.A.™ exam. [For this she took Betafood, see below. She also needed Choline, see Chapter 11, for support for the gallstones.] Luckily with this protocol I never had a crisis. It took longer than I'd expected, but it worked. Now I am able to ingest important oils and move on to the next level of healing."

Now that her body has these EFAs, it can begin to repair her hormonal system. And that subject, which is Crystal's next layer of healing, is addressed in the next chapter, Hormones for Bones.

First, how can these essential fatty acids, the precursors to hormones, be provided, and their assimilation assured?

Protocols

Michael Dobbins, D.C., describes one way health professionals may test for an imbalance in essential fatty acids. After placing a tablet of pure aspirin (acetylsalicylic acid) under someone's tongue, they test an indicator muscle that has been weak. If the muscle strengthens, it indicates a severe ecosanoid system (EFA) imbalance. The test works because the acetyl group in aspirin cuts the production of the whole ecosanoid system, including those that are involved in pain perception.

He adds that when the body indicates such an imbalance, practitioners recommend dietary changes. For example, restricting carbohydrates, as recommended in *Dr. Atkins' New Diet Revolution*, is the fastest way to rebalance the ecosanoid system. Restricting carbohydrates quickly balances brain chemistry, he says, which allows neurotransmitters to get going again.

Dr. Dobbins emphasizes that fatty acids are the optimum food, "the big log on the fire that keeps you warm all night," whereas carbohydrates are "like kindling". When carbohydrates and fats are consumed at the same time, the body deals first with the one more readily oxidized, the carbohydrate, and stores the fat in triglyceride form. "If you then eat more carbohydrates, the body doesn't get back to burning the triglyceride it stored. So the problem was never fat, it was not getting back to the fat to burn it." The solution, he says, is to get on a high fat high protein ketogenic diet immediately in severe cases. He reports that "one woman came in to his office with triglycerides at 1400, immediately went on such a diet, and her levels fell to 200 in 48 hours."[32] Practitioners may also recommend supplementation with black currant seed oil and wheat germ oil.

However, when the liver has been shut down for a long time, reactivating it to carry out its role in EFA metabolism can be difficult. For this problem, Super Eff (see below) is often recommended. It provides EFAs that don't require the liver to break them down. When the liver recovers, it will again be able to produce its own EFAs.

Resupplying the body with essential fatty acids can improve bone health dramatically, and in the process, may also improve conditions such as eczema, P.M.S., sterility, poor wound healing, arthritis, mood swings, seizure disorders, hormone balance and cancer. To supply them, practitioners select among the following:

Linum B6 (SP), which is "organically grown fresh flaxseed oil . . . cold processed [in the right way that preserves their structure] . . . especially high in linolenic acid . . . the most fragile of all oils . . . it goes rancid so easily." It is high in omega 3 fatty acids, which are typically deficient in the American diet. "Flaxseed oil is less likely to be polluted [when organically grown] than fish oils, which are also high in omega 3 fatty acids. An omega 3 deficiency is signified by sticky platelets.[33] Linum B6 contains the vitamin F oils that are the natural antagonist to vitamin D.[34]

Black Currant Seed Oil (SP) is concentrated from cold processed black currant seeds. It has a high quantity of gamma linolenic acid (GLA) and is superior to evening primrose oil as a source of GLAs, a converted form of linolenic acid produced in the liver if it is healthy. It is used up rapidly in people who have inflammatory processes for any reason, whether from working out a lot, from arthritis or a food sensitivity. It's also needed when someone has eczema or very dry skin, for "the body is not converting essential fatty acids into the form that the sebaceous glands under the skin use, which is GLA."[35] Evening primrose oil contains these oils, but in a lesser concentration, making it less potent to rapidly improve bodily stores.

Sesame Seed Oil (SP) contains concentrated "vitamin T", which stands for thrombocyte, which is a blood cell that aids in coagulation of blood. This vitamin is often low in people who have a low thrombocyte count, leukemia, and severe blood conditions, including anemia. In fact, one Midwestern doctor had three children who overcame leukemia by eating six tablespoonfuls of brown sesame butter (which contains high concentrations of the oil) a day.[36] It feeds the bone marrow some of the raw building materials it needs to raise the red blood cell count.

Chlorophyll Complex (SP) is a fat soluble chlorophyll and therefore retains fat soluble nutrients, especially vitamins A, E, F, and K. Chlorophyll Complex is a also a source of Vitamin K, which is involved in the production of fibrin, important in the clotting mechanism. The structure of the chlorophyll molecule is very close to that of hemoglobin, which carries oxygen to the tissues. The main difference is that magnesium is primary in chlorophyll molecules, where iron is present in hemoglobin. Therefore this product is often used for anemia as well as a source of EFAs and of the fat soluble vitamins: A, D, E and K.

States Bruce West, D.C., "It's a rare instance when I do not recommend a Chlorophyll Perle for anyone suffering from kidney stones or osteoporosis. Chlorophyll activates a blood protein called osteocalcin which is critical for the proper formation of bone. Without this activity you cannot build bone [which can lead to osteoporosis] and you develop the chronic formation of calcium oxalate (the major form of kidney stones)." He instructs people to think of this chlorophyll product "when you need to move calcium and other minerals into your bones and out of your kidneys. Chlorophyll is the substance that absorbs trace minerals like boron and molybdenum from soil and gets them into plants. When you consume chlorophyll, you are getting a host of trace minerals and a supreme source of organic magnesium ... the natural balance for calcium, especially when it comes to kidney stones."[37]

He insists on using a chlorophyll product that is truly cold processed, not merely labeled so, which is why he recommends Standard Process. His reasoning is that "there are enzymes in and around the fat soluble chlorophyll molecule that the body needs to build bones from all the other materials which heat processing destroys. If lacking the enzymes, which most people are, they won't build bone properly. Also, few people get a good source of raw fat."[38]

Cataplex F Tablets (SP) are a source of essential polyunsaturated fatty acids, primary arachidonic. The EFAs they contain also include some of arachidonic acid's parents, linoleic and linolenic acid. They help transport calcium from blood to tissues. The EFAs ionize calcium lactate to make it available to the tissues. Cataplex F also contains some protein-bound iodine, and therefore also supports the thyroid, hair, skin and nails. It is used for calcium starvation, calcium assimilation problems, herpes simplex, hypothyroidism, ridged nails, poor hair quality, dry skin, muscle cramps, hypervitaminosis D, sunburn, sun poisoning, sun sensitivity, heat prostration, and prostate problems.

The EFAs in Cataplex F provide the balance to vitamin D, as described previously. The EFAs help spread calcium into the tissues, especially in any condition when the surface (i.e., skin or nails) has become hard or brittle.[39] "For dry bones, Standard Process F Perles are Vitamin F in the oil form (Linum B6), your essential fatty acids."[40] Cataplex F Perles (SP) are similar to Cataplex F tablets except they contain no iodine.

Wheat Germ Oil Perles (SP) can eliminate muscle cramps if they are due to failure of the body to deliver calcium to the muscles. They also contain sex hormone precursors, and are therefore good for hot flashes. This product also contains a vitamin recognized in England, but not in the United States, called "B4". B4 has been known to correct arrhythmias of the heart.[41] Additionally, reports Dr. Versendaal, Wheat Germ Oil is excellent for keeping fallopian tubes and the vas deferens healthy, as it helps keep these tubes from collapsing. It's also used to support scar tissue repair. Some practitioners suggest rubbing it directly into the scar tissue.

Super-EFF (SP) is used to provide arachidonic acid when the liver cannot produce it in the normal way from breaking down essential fatty acids. It provides EFA breakdown products directly for people whose condition is severely degenerated, as in muscular dystrophy or multiple sclerosis.

Betafood (SP) provides nutritional support to aid in the digestion and absorption of essential fatty acids. It is designed to flush the entire route through which bile flows and thus eliminate toxins brought to the liver to be filtered out. If bile gets too thick, it can't flow easily, which indicates that fat metabolism is deficient. It contains concentrated beet juice to help decongest the liver, mobilize bile, and provide methyl donors (for fat metabolism). Six Betafood a day has the cleansing power of eating 20 beets a day! It is completely vegetarian.

A F Betafood (SP) contains Betafood with the addition of Cataplex A and Cataplex F, which provide additional support for detoxification.

In acute situations involving gallstones, practitioners often recommend a combination of products every 15 minutes which may include: 10 Choline (see Chapter 11) 10 Betafood, 10 Linum B6 and 1 dropperful of Phosfood (in previous chapter).[42] Protocols for liver support are included in Chapter 11.

Once essential fatty acids are absorbed and metabolized, the body can begin to use their breakdown products to manufacture the substances that regulate the bone bank. These regulators are the powerful hormones, the subject of Chapter 9.

ENDNOTES

1. Dobbins, Ibid.
2. *Taber's*, Ibid., p. L 31.
3. 20/20 Broadcast, ABC Network, Apr. 10, 1998.
4. Balch and Balch, Ibid., p. 51.
5. Balch and Balch, Ibid., p. 51.
6. *Taber's*, Ibid., p. M 59.
7. Kerry Bodmer with Nan Kathryn Fuchs. *Stop Breast Cancer Before It Happens*. Soundview Publications, Inc., 1997, p. 7.
8. Hunter Yost, M.D. *Molecules for the Mind*, Available at: www.azstarnet.com/healthbeat/mole.html.
9. Available at: www.xs4all.nl/hempy/hemp.html.
10. Dobbins, Ibid.
11. Mack, Ibid.
12. Dobbins, Ibid.
13. Anne Louise Gittleman, M.S. *Beyond Pritikin*, Bantam Books, New York, New York, 1989. Available at: www.barleans.com/flax.html.
14. Clinical Reference Guide, Ibid.
15. Dobbins, Ibid.
16. Mary Frost, M.A. *Going Back to the Basics of Human Health, Avoiding the Fads, the Trends and the Bold-Faced Lies*, self-published, February, 1997, p. 28.

17. Yost, Ibid.
18. Dobbins, Ibid.
19. Balch and Balch, Ibid., p. 51. Also available at: www.pathfinder.com/time/magazine/archive/1994/940905/94090.
20. Dobbins, Ibid.
21. Available at: www.cspinet.org/new/olesnatl.html.
22. Versendaal, Seminar, Ibid.
23. Dobbins, Ibid.
24. Royal Lee, D.D.S., Ibid.
25. Mary Frost, M.A. *Going Back to the Basics of Human Health, Avoiding the Fads, the Trends and the Bold-Faced Lies*, self-published, February, 1997, p. 28.
26. Yost, Ibid.
27. Available at: www.pathfinder.com/time/magazine/archive/1994/940905/94090www.
28. Clinical Reference Guide, Ibid., p. 2.
29. Versendaal, Author's Interview, Ibid.
30. Ibid.
31. Ibid.
32. Dobbins, Ibid.
33. Clinical Reference Guide, Ibid., p. 25.
34. Ibid., p. 15.
35. Ibid., p. 7.
36. Ibid., p. 33.
37. West, Ibid., Vol. 15, Issue 7, July 1998, p. 4.
38. West, Ibid., Vol. 15, Issue 7, July 1998, p. 4.
39. Newell, Ibid.
40. Versendaal, Interview, Ibid.
41. Dobbins, Ibid. Also in letters from Royal Lee, private collection, July 21, 1948.
42. Versendaal and Versendaal-Hoezee. Ibid., p. 116.

Regulating the Bank: Hormones for Bones

W hen hormone imbalances are involved in osteoporosis, they carry the medical diagnosis of "Type I" osteoporosis. But hormones may seem a world away from bones. What does one have to do with the other?

Hormones are the governing officers of the bone bank, regulating all its activity. The president of the board is the pituitary gland. It secretes hormones that oversee and direct the activities of all board members, the other endocrine glands. These include adrenals, thyroid, parathyroid, pineal, pancreas, liver, male gonadal (prostate, testes) or female gonadal (ovary, uterus and mammary), duodenum, thymus, and the power behind the scenes, the hypothalamus. Together they set policies and give directives for the bone bank. It is they who hold the power to determine whether to increase, maintain or withdraw deposits. And, hormones are potent substances: they achieve their objectives in very small amounts.

The word 'hormone' is derived from the Greek, meaning arouse or excite. Technically, hormones are chemical substances made in an organ or gland. Once manufactured, though, they are conveyed through the blood to another part of the body. It is at these target sites that they demonstrate their regulatory command, stimulating some activities and reducing others.

Some hormones are more important to the bone bank than others. For example, Dr. Versendaal points out, "Hormones made by the uterus, prostate and parathyroid gland help the bone marrow produce and release all kinds of minerals."[1] Three other hormones control blood calcium levels (parathyroid hormone, dihydroxy-vitamin D, and calcitonin from the thyroid gland). Together they supervise calcium: how much is absorbed by the intestine, excreted through the kidneys, and taken into bones. Meanwhile, still other hormones (parathormone and progesterone) regulate the deposit of calcium into tissues. To produce these hormones, the body requires essential fatty acids (EFAs). Therefore too low a level of EFAs can create hormone imbalances and deregulate the bone bank.

Assuming enough raw materials to make sufficient hormones, each hormone factory or gland raises its own voice on the governing board relative to its particular assignments. In turn, the release of its potent hormonal substances must be timed and integrated with all the others on the board to produce perfect bones. For example, Dr. Versendaal points out, "The ovaries or testicles produce hormones that are stored in the uterus and prostate. The pituitary gland organizes all of them together: the uterus, prostate, testicles, ovaries, parathyroid."[2]

Hormone production problems are all related to each other: if one lags in production, other board members try to cover their buddy's job. For example, if ovaries or testes are removed or malfunctioning, adrenal glands strive to produce the missing sex hormones. According to Dr. Versendaal, "Many people have bodies that are loaded with calcium, but can't do anything with it because the hormones aren't available, because the prostate, or ovaries, or uterus or parathyroid shut down. Those are the glands that metabolize calcium. In case the uterus or prostate quit working, the parathyroid gland backs them up, especially as in women who have or have had anorexia or who have or are currently over-exercising."[3]

One hormone imbalance can effect other hormone factories like one domino falling in a stack of other dominoes. Dan Newell,

N.D., describes what happens: "The pH normalizing glands are the adrenals and thyroids. When these prime regulators of pH balance are affected, they go into overdrive trying to regulate. When that's been going on for some time, and then the menopausal hormone shift is added to the hormone factories' work load, the pituitary enlarges. The pituitary tries to compensate for the lack of ovarian hormones. Most women notice a headache over their left ear."[4] First the adrenals fail because they're overstressed. The thyroid tries to back them up, but gets tired too. Then the pituitary overworks. By the time the hormonal shift of menopause takes place, the whole stack of dominoes can start tumbling down.

Each board member has not only particular allies, but also antagonists who can oppose their activities. To better understand how health practitioners use clinical nutrition to support the hormonal system, a brief introduction to each one is given below. Individually, they reveal their unique contribution to running the bone bank, and therefore to the quest for Perfect Bones.

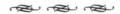

Pituitary. The pituitary is a tiny gland no bigger than a hickory nut that nonetheless wields tremendous power. It sits at the base of the brain, where it chairs the board of bone bank regulators. This leadership position is a well deserved title, for the pituitary produces more hormones than any other gland: hormones that stimulate growth, sexual development, the reproductive cycle, digestion, metabolism, water intake and output, lactation, blood pressure, even labor contractions. For these contributions, it has earned the title "the master gland".

Someone whose pituitary is chronically weak during childhood may grow to be short in stature. But a weak pituitary, says Dr. Versendaal, can also result "in an overacid stomach that nothing seems to help."[5] When it develops an acute weakness, as when it orchestrates the profound hormonal shifts of menopause, for example, it can change metabolism, raise blood pressure, and create disturbances in water intake and output, contributing to hot flashes and night sweats.

The pituitary has particular allies on the governing board— other hormone factory members who will cooperate quickly and supportively when a job needs to be done. The pituitary calls on these particular comrades via particular hormones it manufactures that are specific to these target glands. These best buddies are the thyroid, gonads, mammary and adrenal glands.

But, just in case the pituitary gets out of hand, perhaps too power hungry or not knowing when to quit, there are two other board members who will antagonize it: the pancreas and the duo-denum. If necessary, these two junior board members can cause a complete insurrection!

Thyroid. The thyroid is a horseshoe-shaped gland residing at the front of the neck. It makes a variety of hormones. Bruce West, D.C., refers to it as the "middleman for the way your body balances calcium".[6] According to Dr. Versendaal, the first thyroid hormone, T1, controls the brain's electrical input and charge. T1 is the generator of the brain. When T1 levels are deficient, symptoms can include fatigue, depression, low self-esteem, suicidal tendencies and mental disorders. T1 also controls the brain, eyes, ears, sense of smell. When T1 is weak, Dr. Versendaal says, people are not happy and are tired. Kids with A.D.D. (attention deficit disorder) have tired brains.[7]

The thyroid gland also makes T3, which controls the rhythm of the kidneys. When too little T3 is produced, the person may develop incontinent bowel because they have too many fluids in the body.

T4, Dr. Versendaal points out, controls the rhythm of the heart; therefore deficient levels can cause symptoms such as fatigue, depression, headaches, and cold extremities due to poor circulation. T4 deficiency can also result in goiters, double chins, and symptoms that mimic heart failure.[8]

The relationship of thyroid hormones to bone health is a central one: thyroid hormones are required for bone remodeling to take place. States Alan Gaby, M.D., "Thyroid hormone is one of the triggers for the bone-remodeling cycle, which starts with bone resorption and is followed by new bone formation. If not enough thyroid hormone is present, old bone tends to accumulate—bone that is not necessarily strong or fracture-resistant."[9]

When the thyroid is out of balance, remarks Dr. Versendaal, people can get crabby very quickly. Clinical nutritionist and researcher Dan Newell estimates he has helped several hundred menopausal women rebalance their endocrine systems by providing nutritional support for their thyroids. He says that some women undergoing menopause develop increased thyroid activity, which causes a faster withdrawal rate from the bone bank (a faster turnover in osteoclast activity). Then the parathyroid kicks into high gear too, to get rid of the calcium that got drawn into the blood from the bones. Such women exhibit muscular weakness over the scapula (the upper shoulder area) in the back. The focus of nutritional support is to calm the thyroid down (see protocols below). Probably about 50 to 60% of patients respond to this kind of approach, he adds.[10]

The thyroid's major supporters are the adrenal glands, the pituitary gland, and the gonads (ovaries or testes). The liver is also central to thyroid functioning, since hormones produced by the thyroid are activated in the liver. Chief thyroid antagonists are the thymus, the pancreas, the parathyroid glands and the hormones produced by the breasts in nursing women during lactation.

Parathyroids. The parathyroids are four small glands about the size of a pea that are attached to the thyroid gland. They regulate calcium levels in the blood even more strictly than the pancreas and adrenal glands regulate blood glucose. This regulatory function is lifesaving because proper blood calcium levels are essential for nerve transmission and muscle contraction; and, of

course, the most important nerve transmissions and muscle contractions of all are those of the heart. The parathyroid gland must
keep blood calcium levels high enough to feed the heart nerves
and muscle first. Then, if enough is left over, it can afford to make
bone bank deposits.

If blood calcium levels are too low, the parathyroids make
withdrawals from the bone bank. They remove calcium from
bones because the calcium needs of the heart and other systems
essential to survival come first. "The parathyroid gland is designed
exclusively for calcium utilization; no other gland is dedicated to
one mineral."[11] The parathyroid system operates so quickly, it can
take calcium and phosphorus out of bones or deposit it back in
fractions of a second.

The hormone produced by the parathyroid glands stimulates
the bone marrow to carry out its various functions, including that
of producing red blood cells. Nutritional support for the parathyroid allows it to release a hormone that stimulates bone bank
deposits to be removed at a faster rate. In other words, it stimulates bone-destroying osteoclast cells.

While it may sound like a bad idea to stimulate cells that
help break down bone, quite the opposite is true. In a healthy
body with healthy bones, all aspects of the bone metabolic cycle
are active. If any part of the bone remodeling cycle is inactive or
sluggish, the stage is set for unhealthy bones. An analogy brings
home the point. Consider what would happen to a body that
could ingest food, but not eliminate any of it. That's what happens to bones at the cellular level if the bone breakdown part of
the cycle doesn't work.

The parathyroids back up their allies, the uterus or prostate,
and cooperate with their friends: the pancreas, liver, and gonads.
Their natural antagonist is the thyroid.

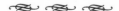

Adrenals. The adrenals are two triangular shaped glands
located one above each kidney. They make over thirty hormones

that constantly shift to mediate differing stress levels. They play a central role in bone health because they participate in maintaining the right mineral balance. But, when they are overactive, chronically turned on, they continue to secrete stress hormones such as cortisol that "attach to bone cells and direct the withdrawal of calcium from the bones."[12] This is actually a favor to the body, for it is via this mechanism that the high, short-term needs for calcium activated during stress are met. But the long-term effect of such adrenal stress hormone overproduction is to thin bones.

But that's not all. Under stress, adrenal hormones decrease calcium absorption in the intestines, and that, too, leads to increased withdrawal of calcium from the bones.[13] It's easy to tell when the adrenals are in a stress response because they secrete epinephrine (also called adrenalin). This hormone makes the heart race, the blood pressure elevate, arterioles constrict, digestion shut down, and glucose be liberated from the liver in preparation to fight, freeze, or flee.

Adrenals go into high gear under the influence of pain, fear, rage or asphyxia (a state of suspended animation due to interference with the oxygen supply of the blood). However, once such threats are over, they can forget to settle down, thus continuing, quietly, to leach calcium deposits from the bone bank. That's one reason why it's so important not to live life on an "adrenaline high". The invisible, bone-robbing cost of chronic stress can cause complete bone bank failure. One early symptom of adrenal weakening due to prolonged stress is that the body fills up with fluid. A warning sign of possible adrenal overload is puffy bags under the eyes.

Adrenals also produce other, male-type sex hormones (including DHEA) that affect bone health positively. High DHEA levels are correlated with greater bone mineral content, and low levels with low bone mineral content. Therefore, keeping adrenals functioning well is one way to contribute to perfect bones.

But that's not the only reason to keep adrenals happy. "Adrenals are the second backup to the heart after the thyroid."[14] Also, they have some ability to compensate for low sex hormone levels if too little is secreted by the ovaries or testes. That in itself is a major contribution to bone health, particularly after midlife.

Glands that cooperate with the adrenals include the thyroid, gonads and pituitary. Those that antagonize adrenals are the pancreas, duodenum, thymus, gonads and parathyroids.[15]

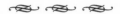

Gonads. Gonadal hormones play a key role in directing calcium metabolism for both women and men. Women's ovaries produce three types of such hormones: estrogens, progesterone and androgens. Estrogen has received a lot of attention for osteoporosis prevention because it increases calcium absorption and slows down or inhibits the rate of calcium withdrawal from the bone bank. However, the bone benefit of ingesting synthetic estrogen after menopause wanes after 3–5 years, John Lee, M.D., points out.[16] He concludes, "The strength of the estrogen-fixed mindset represents a victory of advertising over science."[17] Dr. Lee emphasizes that the crux of the problem is that "healthy, well nourished [ovarian] follicle cells produce a healthy balance of estrogen and progesterone." Malnourished follicles can shut down, requiring nutritional support to produce hormones. Well nourished follicles (or the hormones they produce) are a necessary precondition for preventing or reversing osteoporosis. In men, the male sex hormone testosterone replaces estrogens and is produced by cells in the testes.

Progesterone is important to bone because it both stimulates the rate of bone bank deposits and helps limit withdrawals. As such, progesterone is possibly the most important hormone for healthy bones. A recent study in *The New England Journal of Medicine* reports that osteoporosis occurs in athletes to the degree that they become progesterone deficient. This hormone "acts directly on bone by engaging an osteoblast receptor or indirectly through competition for a glucocorticoid osteoblast receptor...the normal ovulatory cycle looks like a natural bone-activating, coherence cycle."[18] "Progesterone restores osteoblast function."[19]

Men's bodies also make progesterone, which is then is turned into testosterone by the testes. Whether in men or in women, "Like progesterone, testosterone can stimulate new bone formation, increase bone density, and a lack of it can cause osteoporosis."[20] Although men's hormone shifts are not as dramatic as women's during menopause, nonetheless, during men's corollary phase, sometimes called "andropause" or "viropause" or "manopause", testosterone levels do drop, exposing men, too, to the risks of developing sick bones. Restoration of testosterone levels reverses these deleterious effects, even if they are a result of treatment with glucocorticoid drugs.[21]

Indeed, many people have inadequate or imbalanced levels of gonadal hormones. One reason is radiation, another is starvation. For example, people who keep themselves on a strict low-fat diet, with too few essential fatty acids (EFAs), don't have enough of these building blocks to make sex hormones. Progesterone is formed predominantly in the ovary, to a lesser extent by the adrenals, and to some extent, by nerves. It is formed in these tissues from cholesterol. Thus, people who suffer from anorexia also eventually stop producing the sex hormones necessary for bone health due to lack of these EFAs and other nutrients. Ultimately they become amenorrheic (without a period), and the longer they remain so, the more severely their bones are damaged. The same effect occurs in women who overexercise: their bones deteriorate when their bodies can no longer produce the sex hormones they need for bone health.

Another major contributor to gonadal hormone inadequacy is surgical removal of these hormone factories. For women, each year "well over half a million women in the United States undergo surgical ovary removal.[22] "Thirty-four percent of U.S. women will have had their uterus removed by age 66. It's the second-most common surgery performed.[23] In terms of numbers, that translates to "650,000 or more hysterectomies per year performed in the United States."[24] Of these, some 1,200 die from the procedure.[25] In Britain, more than 1,000 women per week undergo hysterectomy, usually in their early forties, a surgery which contributes to loss of bone health and the onset of osteoporosis.[26] Even when only the uterus is removed, the remaining ovaries often fail to function after the surgery.[27]

For men who lack testosterone, for example "men castrated either surgically or chemically, [they] will experience accelerated osteoporosis within two to three years. Such a condition happens, for example, in the treatment of prostate cancer."[28] The current incidence of prostate cancer is one man in six. And the number one cancer among men 20–34 is testicular.[29]

Hypogonadal (low sex hormone producing) men require sex hormone support to prevent osteoporosis for the same reasons women require hormone replacement.[30] And one key reason is that they will lose bone mass without it. This support can easily be provided free of unwanted effects using the vegetarian sex hormone protocol (see below). Still, they are often denied it.

An often overlooked part of the reproductive hormonal system is the hormones produced by the mammary glands. Unfortunately, few studies have been conducted about their role. As far back as 1932, Henry Harrower, M.D., who wrote the seminal work of that time on the endocrine system, pointed out that the mammary glands secrete many substances science was not yet aware of.[31] Michael Dobbins, D.C., adds, "Many women's systems won't balance without adding mammary, which often acts as the catalyst to open up the [hormonal] system."[32]

Hypothalamus. The hypothalamus is a key regulatory player for all the members of the bone bank governing board. If the pituitary is the power on the throne, then the hypothalamus is the power behind the throne. It lies deep in the brain where it exerts control over the secretions of the other endocrine glands, especially "stop" and "go" messages to the nervous system. It even regulates the chair of the board, the pituitary. It also monitors sex hormone levels and their bodily effects. And it acts as a "pacemaker" to drive biological rhythms, including the sleep and wake cycle. Dr. John Lee likens it to a giant analog computer complex that can make and send signals to the pituitary gland. It can even control the autonomic nervous system (involuntary) balance and modulate the immune system. It even influences emotional states and the responses the body makes to them.

The functions of the hypothalamus gland are influenced by pain and by smell, by digestive functions in the intestines, and by concentrations of nutrients, electrolytes, water and hormones. It also responds to messages from the limbic or emotional brain. This input into the endocrine system by the nervous system is one of the reasons all the hormonal regulators in action are referred to as "neuroendocrine function".

Hypothalamic operations are interfered with by stress, especially emotional pressure, and by poor diet—especially protein deficiency and pollutants, including synthetic progestins and birth control pills. Such deficiencies and pollutants, says John Lee, M.D., create hypothalamic imbalances that can lead to "decreased immune response, decreased adrenal response, sleep disorders, peptic ulcers, depression, anxiety, panic, rage, learning disorders, and hormone disorders."[33] The hypothalamus' functions can be brought into check by two of its main antagonists: neurotransmitters and pituitary feedback.

Hormones indeed play a critical role in bone health. What might hormonal imbalances look like in one person? One 81-year-old grandfather has such a story to tell. John G. reports, "When I was 75, I had some symptoms, including loss of bladder control. I went to the doctor and found out I had prostate cancer. First I had radiation for several months. Then I began to complain about my hip. So they took an x-ray and found out yes, it was metastasized to the bone. The doctor decided my cancer was feeding on testosterone, so [to get rid of the testosterone] I was given a choice of chemical or surgical approach. I chose surgical, a total orchiectomy, complete removal of the testicles. I didn't like the odds for the chemical approach: 15 months to live.

He continues, "Then I became interested in the alternative approach. A New York doctor wrote a book about macrobiotics, and I started [reading] it right after I recovered from surgery. Then I found out it [the cancer] was metastasized to the bone and they'd given me 16 months to live. My daughter suggested I get tested by a C.R.A.™ practitioner. I got tested by Mary Jane Mack, R.N. I went on the protocols for yeast and virus. I took the protocols and in two and a quarter months happened to have another appointment back with the urologist. After doing some tests, he came back in shock; my PSA [prostate-specific antibody] level had dropped to zero. I talked with the doctors about these alternatives but they took the position that there was nothing in their medical practice that would lead to recommending C.R.A.™, but since it was an alternative practice, try it. Then when I got the wonderful test results, the doctor wouldn't admit it was from the C.R.A.™, but I thought it was. That was three years ago, and I've had two zero PSAs since."

Since the surgery, he says he's "developed a stoop and am shrinking in height. I can't drink out of a normal cup for coffee because my head tilts too far forward. I have to put my head way back. I've had muscle tension a long time. I was once evaluated by a psychiatrist; his conclusion was I had a psychoneurosis tension state. I had no muscle problems until I got my sciatic condition. In my right leg I have to be very careful in how I move my leg a certain way, I get the feeling of precramping." He's also noticed tooth pain. He feels "the stoop and losing height happened some before the surgery, but after it happened much faster.

I'm eighty-one years and a quarter now; I was seventy-eight when I had the surgery."

He continues, "I haven't taken any hormones after the surgery. I talked to my urologist about some chemical replacement and he said he preferred I not take any out of concern I might have a flare-up. I'd had bone cancer at the time of the operation. I'd prefer to have some sort of treatment or replacement of testosterone lost by surgery. I have so much fatigue, and that's very limiting. I need morning naps and afternoon naps and naps before bed. I also have a softening of my muscular structure. I don't believe I increased breast size but I got a lot more flabby. Then, two years ago, I started to have symptoms of Parkinson's."

I tested John using C.R.A.™ during this interview and found his osteoporosis reflex did indeed test weak, and also that he was very weak for sex hormone protocols and oils. Despite his PSAs staying so low, and his symptoms of osteoporosis, his urologist has not recommended any hormone replacement. However, with the last exam, John reports, his urologist finally "recommended a diet which included low fat and soy and a lot of what's recommended by macrobiotics. He even said he's on it himself."

John clearly demonstrates the need for the concentrated nutritional protocols that would support his hormonal system. However, the form of nutritional support needed to help restore hormonal balance is highly individual. John needs sex hormone support and essential fatty acids. Maureen Schaub decided to find out what she needed.

Maureen, a beautician and mother of two children, already had a dowager's hump and back pain at age 33. She says, "I was worried about not getting enough calcium, and my back was hurting. I got inflamed discs a lot in my upper back, which I think is due to the stress of my profession, having my arms up all the time. My grandma on my dad's side had osteoporosis, and that's always concerned me. Even before my profession I was hunched over. I am intolerant both to lactose and milk protein, my digestive system is very sensitive. The older I get the more back problems I have. Also my energy level wasn't good, so I decided to give C.R.A.™ a try and see what it could do with me."

"First I had an infection in one of my lungs from my work environment, all the chemicals I'd been around, so I took Parotid (SP, see Chapter 11). I still take a low maintenance dose based on the amount of chemicals I'm around that day."

Such chemicals can indeed deplete bone bank deposits. But even more significant has been her need for various forms of hormonal support. The first of these was her thyroid, for which she took 6 Thytrophin PMG (SP) and 3 Organic Iodine (SP). She explains, "I started having thyroid problems when I was 13. My thyroid was so enlarged it came out to where my chin is. The doctor sent me to a thyroid specialist. He wanted my body to try to develop on its own, so he didn't give me anything. So I took kelp on my own. I don't know if it helped or not. When I had my first child, my daughter, my thyroid whacked out." She was given DES to guarantee that she wouldn't miscarry. She adds, "My mom took DES too, to guarantee that she wouldn't miscarry me."

Thyroid support was central to restoring Maureen's hormonal balance in preparation for bone repair. But three other hormone factories needed nutrition too, probably from trying to back up a weak thyroid all those years. Over time, she has also needed support for her pituitary, for which she has taken either 2 Pituitrophin (SP) or 2 Symplex F; for sex hormones, for which she took 3 Ovex and 2 Catalyn; and adrenals, for which she took B6-Niacinamide (SP).

After her hormone system came back into balance, she began addressing nutritional needs for bone repair. For one, she needed a blood builder, for which she took 1 e-Poise a day. She also needed gallbladder support, and she was put on 3 Betafood per day.

Then, she says, "I was taking Calcium Lactate [to supplement her calcium intake] but I would still hold my body tense. So Laura (her C.R.A.™ practitioner) put me on Cal-Ma Plus (which is calcium lactate plus parathyroid support), and also the flax seed pill [Linum B6, SP] to help it absorb better. I started noticing a difference within a week, especially my shoulder area and back, being able to relax better. And the pain subsided. I still take it, and feel like I'll take it forever. I'd rather, knowing I don't use dairy products. I want to make sure I'm in better health.

"Since I've been on the Cal-Ma Plus my discs inflame far less often, and far less severely when they do. Before, my disc would be inflamed quite often, but now it's only during the times I'm really busy at work. If I don't take the flax seed oil with it, I do notice a difference…a little stiffer feeling. The oil helps it get into the system better. I took three Cal-Ma Plus a day originally, and now take two or three each night. If I go totally off it, if I forget, I feel the difference in my body. I've been taking it now for four months.

"Now I give my kids flax seed oil and calcium lactate when they have growing pains, and it takes the growing pains away. Their bones are growing so fast. Doing it the natural way is so much better than man-made drugs that suppress the problem. The clinical nutrition gets to the core of the problem, which is important to me."[34]

Protocols

The following hormonal protocols help feed the body what it needs so it can make its own hormones and bring them into balance.

PITUITARY:

Symplex F (SP, for females) or *Symplex M* (SP, for males) (6 a day for 3 months) is indicated for multiple hormone imbalances, including hypothalamic. These products contain nutrition that supports the pituitary, thyroid, adrenals and ovaries or testes. It also contains chlorophyll (see below). It may especially be needed after the hormonal shifts of menopause or prepuberty. Because pituitary support can help balance the entire hormonal system, *Symplex F or M* can benefit the bone bank in all the ways discussed above. An additional advantage is that it can help balance mood swings, and may improve sexual responsiveness in both men and women. Many practitioners are also using it to support brain growth and functioning in children, including those with cerebral palsy and/or mental retardation.

For-Til B12 (SP, 3 a day for 3 months) is often recommended for hormone support because it is rich in vitamin E and other factors needed to make sex hormones. It contains tillandsia, found in Spanish moss. It is excellent for people who are fatigued and worn out.[35]

Catalyn (SP, 3 to 6 a day) was the first product made by Royal Lee when he started Standard Process. His chief goal was to provide nutritional support for all the endocrine glands. It acts as a biochemical catalyst. It contains a myriad of multiple vitamins, trace minerals and enzymes. (See also Chapter 7.)

Pituitrophin PMG (SP, 2–6 a day for 3 months) is used for general pituitary support, and when the pituitary is hyperactive (hyperpituitary). It supports people with metabolic disorders, delayed healing, gastrointestinal ulcers, and nervous symptoms. It is high in trace minerals, B12 and vitamin E complex. It is combined with Neuroplex and E-Manganese (see below) for a weak or low functioning gland (hypopituitary).

E-Manganese, (SP, 4 a day) supports the anterior pituitary's high demand for manganese and vitamin E complex.

THYROID:

Thytrophin (SP, 3–9 a day) contains a combination of nutrition designed to provide general support to the thyroid gland. If the thyroid is overworking, Antronex may be added. Also, Thytrophin may be combined with Allorganic Trace Minerals B12, to support slowing the thyroid.[36] If it is underworking, Betafood and Niacinamide B6 may be added.

Min-Tran (SP, 6 a day) (short for mineral tranquilizers) is a source of alkaline ash minerals combined with calcium lactate. These are nutrients that support thyroid T1 function. Up to 15 a day are sometimes recommended for people who are very tired until their tiredness is gone.

Organic Minerals (SP, see Chapter 7) are a different blend of minerals also used for thyroid support.

Organic Iodine (SP, 1–3 per *week*) supports the thyroid by providing protein-bound iodine. It is used at a dose of 1 per day to control hot flashes in menopausal women. Dr. Versendaal also recommends it for "people at computers all day; they need iodine to lubricate the body."[37]

Iodomere (SP, 3–6 a day) is also a source of protein-bound iodine in combination with sea minerals. It contains portions of the sea conch. It gives nutritional support to a sluggish thyroid, especially when low thyroid function is associated with fluid retention which results in swelling and wastes backing up in the kidneys.

A-C Carbamide (SP) supports the thyroid function having to do with the osmotic transfer of body fluids through cell walls; therefore it is used for water retention problems related to low thyroid function. (SP, 3–12 per day) (See also Chapter 10.)

PARATHYROID:

Cal-Ma Plus (SP) contains Calcium Lactate combined with desiccated parathyroid gland to enhance the absorption of calcium. Desiccated products are those made from a concentrate of the whole gland. It is designed specifically for parathyroid support. Supporting the parathyroid gland can sometimes unlock the door to healing bones. Says Dr. Versendaal, "Sometimes you put them on support for all these other glands and nothing works, but then you address the parathyroid gland and they start healing."[38] Cal-Ma Plus is also used when the person is unable to metabolize iron. If the parathyroid is underactive, 1 Cal-Ma Plus may be combined with 6 Cataplex F Perles a day for 12 weeks; then 2 Cataplex F Perles, 1 Cal-Ma Plus per day. If the parathyroid is overactive, 6 Cataplex D may be substituted for the Cataplex F.[39]

Cataplex F (SP, 3–6 a day) (see also previous chapter on essential fatty acids) is also used for parathyroid support. Dr. Versendaal explains, "somebody with a prostate problem or uterus problem needs to address the parathyroid gland with F Perles as a backup to the uterus or prostate. So if they have cancer, or had radiation or had these organs removed, use this as a backup. The F perles help the parathyroid gland produce parathyroid hormone."[40] Cataplex F is also used to calm down the thyroid because the unsaturated fatty acids it contains make iodine more diffusible, available for use by the thyroid so it can balance itself.

Cataplex D (SP, 6 a day) is used to balance an overactive parathyroid gland (hyperparathyroid). It is rarely needed, as most people have enough vitamin D in their diets or make sufficient quantities on exposure to sunlight.

Desiccated Parathyroid (SP) draws calcium from the reserves and puts it in the blood. Thus, states Michael Dobbins, D.C., "it is NOT used for osteoporosis. Instead, it's good for muscle cramps, tetany [muscle spasms often related to parathyroid deficiency], short-term muscle cramping."[41] He adds, "The *only* reason to use it long-term is if the parathyroids have been removed."

ADRENAL GLANDS:

B6 Niacinamide (SP, 3–12 per day) contains adrenal hormone precursors that support the bone bank. It also contains nutrients central to the making of connective tissue. Michael Dobbins, D.C., explains that proteins and trace minerals bind to the organic collagen net. The production of these proteins is greatly aided by vitamin B6.[42] It is used as nutritional support for adrenal insufficiency.

One of the symptoms of weak adrenal glands is a low level of DHEA (short for dehydroepiandrosterone), a hormone produced naturally by the adrenal glands and also by the ovaries. Some studies have concluded that DHEA increases bone strength. Therefore it has been recommended as part of the treatment for osteoporosis. Dr. Alan Gaby explains that DHEA is the only hormone which appears capable of both inhibiting bone bank withdrawals (bone resorption) and stimulating bone bank deposits, or bone formation. High DHEA levels and higher density of the spinal bones are associated. Women with osteoporosis have been shown to have lower levels of DHEA at all ages than those without osteoporosis.[43]

However, Bruce West, D.C., cautions, "dabbling in hormones has a cascade effect . . . you are being sold a hormone product that simply masks a laboratory finding of low DHEA levels. And worse, it leaves the more serious condition developing and tinkers with the balance of your adrenal gland hormones . . . Don't complicate matters by taking DHEA supplements"[44] He adds that since DHEA can be converted into estrogen and testosterone in the body, it may be "the kiss of death" for a woman prone to estrogen-induced cancer or a man prone to testosterone-induced cancer of the prostate.[45] Michael Dobbins, D.C., concurs: "For DHEA: if you need it, make it, don't buy it. Support your adrenals. Feed them. Low DHEA is adrenal insufficiency."[46]

Drenamin (SP, 3–9 per day) is a combination of nutrients to support weak adrenal glands. Because it is made from animal adrenal glands, it may be recommended for people whose adrenals are chronically fatigued or for those who have low blood sugar and low blood pressure. It is used short term when the adrenals need a rest before starting to function at a higher level. It functions as a quick start spark for people with acute adrenal exhaustion, and is not used long term except for people in professional sports.

Drenatrophin PMG (SP) contains the nutritional substrate adrenal glands need for repair. It is often recommended for people who demonstrate respiratory weaknesses or allergies.

Whole Desiccated Adrenal (SP, 2 a day) is often used short term when rapid adrenal support is needed, as in shock or sudden, severe stress. It may be used for 2 or 3 weeks, but not long term.[47] Its use is not recommended for more than 30 days.[48]

GONADAL:

Phytoestrogens are a group of compounds found in plants that can influence the body's own estrogen activity. They can both provide precursors so the body can manufacture its own estrogen, or act as a weak estrogen. Hundreds of plants contain these compounds, including red clover, licorice, Dong Quai, soy beans, flaxseeds, black cohosh and alfalfa. Animals have been known to graze selectively on these plants to enhance or diminish fertility.[49] They are a relatively safe way to affect estrogen activity in the body.

Progesterone and testosterone are equivalent hormones when it comes to new bone formation. Recently three creams have become available. The first of these is *testosterone propionate ointment* cream obtainable as a prescription formulated by a pharmacy. It provides testosterone when levels are low.

The second is natural *progesterone cream* made from Mexican yams. Science has known about this source of natural progesterone since 1949.[50] This natural product has been shown to completely halt women's osteoporosis in its tracks, reversing bone bank withdrawals and restoring bone without the dangerous side effects of synthetic progestins. Progesterone cream has also had encouraging results with men, but has not yet been scientifically studied.[51] Progesterone cream is especially used for follicular inadequacy. The answer to this condition, John Lee, M.D., states, "is good nutrition, avoidance of toxins, and proper supplementation, when indicated for hormone balance, or real, honest-to-God, natural progesterone."[52] Lee adds, "It is a mystery to me why synthetic progestins are recommended when the natural progesterone is available, cheaper and safer."[53]

The following are concentrated nutritional protocols that "work at a deeper level than ProGest® Cream."[54] They provide the nutritional support to organs so they can manufacture their own progesterone.

Utrophin (SP, 1–3 per day) is an extract that promotes healthy tissue and balances the hormone production and storage in the uterus.[55] Some practitioners have reported this product (or, for men, Prost-X) having for some people an anti-depressant effect similar to the drug Prozac, which also works on the hormonal system. "The drug masks what's really going on; it takes care of superficial pain or discomfort but underneath is still the same problem."[56]

Prost-X (SP, 3–6 per day) is an aqueous prostate extract that helps transport calcium into bones. If the prostate lacks calcium, it will become enlarged.[57]

Ovex (SP, 3–6 per day) supports female androgen production. It aids calcium assimilation, supports the ovaries and provides vitamin E for steroid hormone production. It was developed to stop heavy menstrual bleeding. It contains enzymes that help the body make progesterone as opposed to estrogen. When progesterone levels are too low, periods last too long; in an estrogen deficiency, they are too short.[58] It has demonstrated good clinical results in women who had difficulty getting pregnant or who have hot flashes, PMS or depression, as it supports weak ovaries.

Orchex (SP, 3–9 per day) provides nutritional support for the production and balance of sex hormones. It is used in acute situations for people whose hormone production is so far off balance that they're about to blow their stack! It's also given to women for menopausal hypertension, and to men with hypertension.[59]

HYPOTHALAMUS:

Hypothalamus PMG (SP, 1–3 per day) is often recommended when hormonal imbalance is accompanied by depression and disturbances in the thirst and satiation centers. It's for people who say, "I don't get satisfied! I eat a meal and still want to continue eating."[60]

Neuroplex (4 a day for 3 months) provides nutritional support for the hypothalamus so it can coordinate the activity of the endocrine system with that of the nervous system. It is also used to support people with brain stem injury, children who can't talk, stutterers, autism; any situation in which there is evidence of difficulty processing thoughts, with flow of information. It is also used for people with spinal cord injuries.

Symplex F or M and For-Til B12 are also used for nutritional support for the hypothalamus (see above).

VEGETARIAN:

Vegetarian protocols for all the various hormone systems are built around providing essential fatty acid precursors; therefore protocols for general hormonal support as well as for pituitary, ovarian, uterine, testicular, prostatic, and mammary hormones are similar:

3 Black Currant Seed Oil
3 Chlorophyll Complex Perles
3 Linum B6
3 Wheat Germ Oil Perles

ADRENAL:

5 Black Currant Seed Oil
3 Chlorophyll Complex Perles

THYROID:

T1: 6 Min-Tran
T4: 2 Organic Minerals per day, or
1–3 Organic Iodine,
3 Linum B6,
3 Chlorophyll,
3 RNA
T4 1/2: 1–3 Organic Iodine,
3 Linum B6,
3 Chlorophyll Complex
3 RNA
T3: 3–9 A-C Carbamide.

Balancing the hormonal system has a variety of effects, depending on the person. For people who are devoid of the food precursors necessary to guard the hormones from oxidation, a fatty acid imbalance may next be revealed (Point Four). Maureen

Schaub's next layer of healing was minerals (Point Two). Or, on the other hand, notes Mary Jane Mack, R.N., "it can go back to blood quality [lack of nutrition in the blood, see Point Six] because the body has nothing to work with."[61]

For me, getting my hormones balanced opened the floodgates to allow deposits to return to the bone bank. That proved to be the last crucial link in creating abundant bone bank mineral deposits. The minerals poured back into my bones, and I could feel my strength returning, not weekly or daily, but hourly. So rapidly were my bones now able to heal, that I had to carry minerals with me and take them throughout the day to meet the demand. But it was worth it! I became able to sit, to carry things, to move swiftly. And, I developed stamina! Instead of dragging, my body demanded to be active, to move, a subject of the next chapter.

ENDNOTES

1. Versendaal, Author's Interview, Ibid.
2. Versendaal, Author's Interview, Ibid.
3. Versendaal, Author's Interview, Ibid.
4. Newell, Author's Interview, Ibid.
5. Versendaal and Versendaal-Hoezee, Ibid, p. 53.
6. West, Author's Interview, Summer 1998.
7. Versendaal and Versendaal-Hoezee, Ibid, p. 32.
8. Ibid, p. 32.
9. Gaby, Ibid, p. 231.
10. Newell, Author's Interview, Ibid.
11. Clinical Reference Guide, Ibid., p. 10.
12. Brown, Ibid., p. 183.
13. Brown, Ibid., pp. 183-4.
14. Versendaal and Versendaal-Hoezee, Ibid., p. 33.
15. Henry R. Harrower, M.D. *Practical Endocrinology*, Second Edition, Lee Foundation for Nutritional Research, Milwaukee, Wisc., 1957, p. 46.

16. Lee, *Natural Progesterone, the Multiple Roles of a Remarkable Hormone*, p. 53.
17. Lee, Ibid, p. 55.
18. J. C. Prior. "Progesterone as a Bone-Trophic Hormone" in *Endocrine Reviews*, Vol. 11, No. 2, May 1990, p. 386.
19. Lee, Ibid., p. 69.
20. John Lee, M.D., with Virginia Hopkins, *What Your Doctor May Not Tell You about Menopause, The Breakthrough Book on Natural Progesterone*. Warner, New York, 1996, p. 79.
21. I. R. Reid, and others. "Testosterone Therapy in Glucocorticoid-Treated Men." *Archives of Internal Medicine*, 156, no. 11 (June 1996): pp. 1173-7.
22. Brown, Ibid, p. 188.
23. Jim Paterson. "Is there "male menopause"? in *USA Weekend*, Jan. 2-4, 1998, p. 16.
24. John Lee with Hopkins, Ibid., p. xvii.
25. Bodmer, "Health Secrets for Women Only" Ibid., October 1998, p. 7.
26. Dover, Ibid.
27. Brown, Ibid., p. 188.
28. John Lee with Hopkins, *What Your Doctor May Not Tell You about Menopause, The Breakthrough Book on Natural Progesterone*, Ibid., p. 128.
29. Paterson, Ibid., p. 16.
30. Medical Data Exchange (MDX), available at: http://www.oclc.org/oclc/man/mdxhd/titlebar.htm
31. Harrower, Ibid., 133.
32. Michael Dobbins, D.C., Ibid.
33. Lee with Hopkins, *What Your Doctor May Not Tell You about Menopause*, Ibid., p. 110.
34. Maureen Schaub, Author's Interview.
35. Clinical Reference Guide, Ibid., p. 21.
36. Standard Process Training Session, see also symptom survey evaluation form.
37. Versendaal, Author's Interview, Ibid.

38. Versendaal, Author's Interview, Ibid., and Clinical Reference Guide, p. 10.

39. Versendaal, Author's Interview, Ibid.

40. Ibid.

41. Dobbins, Ibid.

42. Ibid.

43. Gaby, Ibid., pp. 163-165.

44. West, Ibid., Vol. 15, Issue 2, p. 4.

45. West, Ibid., Vol 14, Issue 7, p. 3.

46. Dobbins, Ibid.

47. Clinical Reference Guide, Ibid., p. 2.

48. Training Session, Ibid. Also Symptom Survey Form.

49. Debbie Moskowitz, N.D. "Phytoestrogens—An Exciting Alternative", reprinted from *Natural Solutions*, Vol. IV, Issue 4, Fall 1996.

50. William Campbell Douglass, M.D. "Say Goodbye to Illness" in *Health Breakthroughs*, Fall 1997, p. 12.

51. John Lee with Hopkins, *What Your Doctor May Not Tell You About Menopause, The Breakthrough Book on Natural Progesterone*. Ibid., p. 78.

52. Lee with Hopkins, Ibid., p.35.

53. Lee with Hopkins, Ibid., p. 47.

54. Mack, Ibid.

55. Versendaal and Versendaal-Hoezee, Ibid., p. 46.

56. Mack, Ibid.

57. Clinical Reference Guide, Ibid., p. 31.

58. Clinical Reference Guide, Ibid., p. 30.

59. Clinical Reference Guide, Ibid., p. 28.

60. Newell, Ibid.

61. Mack, Ibid.

CHAPTER TEN

Stimulating Deposit Activity: Muscles and Metabolism

The very essence of life is activity. Because bones are living tissue, to stay healthy, they require both voluntary, energetic movement and the involuntary movements of the metabolic cycle. Voluntary activities create demand, which stimulates bones to respond. Exercise both activates the bone bank deposit process (because bone-building osteoclast cells increase their activity) and reduces bone bank withdrawals (because the bone-destroying cells slow their activity). This state of affairs—receiving lots of deposits and reducing withdrawals—is indeed a happy one for bones.

Without the catalyst of exercise, bones become weak. Jack Malka, M.D., describes what happens when bones are at rest and not being asked to do much. For example, "when normal bones are in a cast, they are protected from mechanical stress... Therefore they don't need as much strength. They remodel and become weaker than before, reducing the mass of that bone. Once out of the cast, when additional stresses are placed they will again remodel and increase strength until they return to normal."

The rapid decrease in bone mass that results from immobilization is a long known fact. It's been especially well documented in people requiring bed rest and those with some regional form of immobilization such as partial or total paralysis. In fact, people who don't move are in danger of having their mineral deposits made, not in their bones, but in their soft tissues such as arteries, or formed into stones which can lodge in the kidneys.[1]

Gravity is essential to keeping bones healthy. Astronauts in outer space lose bone mass, not because of immobilization, but because of lack of gravity. The Skylab astronauts, for example, stayed highly active but still withstood bone losses comparable to bedridden people. In a weightless environment, their bones didn't have the demand that carrying their own body weight creates on earth to keep them healthy.

Exercise promotes healthy bones because biochemically, the bones go after calcium in response to weight bearing. Backpacking, for example, where bones undergo mechanical loading, stimulates bone bank deposit activity (osteoblasts). It is likely that hormones (in particular, somatotropin) give the "marching orders" to these bone-building cells.

What this means is that putting demands on the skeleton via exercise is a non-negotiable part of the quest for perfect bones.

Voluntary Movement

Kinds of Exercise. No doubt, any movement is better than none. Studies have demonstrated that some non weight-bearing exercises may be helpful to bones. But not all exercise is equal in building bone mass. The most effective bone health-promoting activities are those that make muscles work against gravity or resistance: aerobic movement, weightbearing, and resistance exercises. "Pulling of the muscles on the skeleton through exercise and activity keeps the skeleton strong and the bone responsive to the message to rebuild properly."[2]

For example, people who play tennis have heavier bones in the arm they use to serve the ball than in their non-serving side. And long-distance runners' spines are more substantial than those of people who rarely exercise.[3] "Bone tissue is dynamic and, as it is worked, it increases its absorption of the minerals that give it density."[4]

As part of their osteoporosis prevention project, the Colorado Department of Health recommends the following activities as best for bones: walking, stair climbing, hiking, jogging, skiing, cross-country ski machines, stair-step machines, dancing, aerobic dancing, treadmill walking, weight training, tennis, step classes and gardening. They add that "swimming or bicycling are probably also helpful, especially when swimmers use fins and paddles, and bicyclers ride up hills." They conclude that "it is important to exercise both the upper and lower parts of the body to strengthen all of the bones."[5]

If you like to swim and want to keep that as your primary bone building activity, you might be interested in the results of the broadest study yet of bone density, conducted at Australia's Edith Cowan University. "Doctors surveyed 60 female athletes and found that those who had engaged in high-impact sports for 20–30 years had much stronger bones than those who swam." These findings imply that swimmers in their twenties and thirties might want to start now to introduce some weight bearing activity into their exercise programs.

Who Can Benefit. To reap the bone benefits of exercise, apparently the best course of action would have been to be active in childhood, before age 20, when most peak bone mass develops. For example, of 155 women studied in Bath, England, those who "recalled doing a great deal of walking when they were youngsters had developed the strongest thigh bones", which are the strongest bones in the body.[6]

But if you led a sedentary childhood, and even a sedentary adulthood up to this point, don't despair. It's never too late to reap the benefits of activity. Indeed, exercise all through life is an important tool to prevent osteoporosis. Men and women age 50 to 70 who exercise regularly have been shown to have 30% denser bones than their non-exercising counterparts.

How, then, to begin?

To Safely Begin. Even though weight bearing exercise provides the penultimate benefit to bones, that may be more than many osteoporosis sufferers can manage. That was true for me at the low point of my bone loss. At first I couldn't even walk because I'd get injured and have to spend a long, inactive time recovering. Yet I knew that becoming active was essential. Luckily my health care professionals advised me to stay under what I could do; in other words, to proceed, but not to push myself. The key for my beginning safely was getting into water where I could move slowly and carefully with the water supporting me. From there, I slowly graduated to being able to walk, then carry a backpack, then hike, bike and use weights. Gradually, my body relearned to be active and to stay that way.

If you are fairly inactive now, you may feel defeated to think you have to do 30–45 minutes of aerobic activity nearly every day, as many experts recommend. If that goal sounds impossible, you may want to start with the aim of increasing what you now do. After all, your body wants to move—that's how it is designed.

Grown-ups have to exert a lot of effort to get kids to sit still. Being in motion is the natural state of the body, and a healthy body continues naturally to want activity. If supported properly with good nutrition and healthy activity, it will slowly regain its ability to do all kinds of things. Eventually your body can return to that free, childlike state, when you want to move and you can do so joyfully!

To get to that state of recovery, Barbara Drinkwater, an exercise physiologist and one of the country's leading bone density experts, recommends that you increase duration and intensity of exercise by no more than 10% per week.[7]

Don't let yourself get stopped by not knowing which activity you should do. Think about what your body is currently able to do and what would be fun. Anything is better than nothing. Do something, even two minutes worth. Then congratulate yourself for it. Refuse to allow room for a negative turn of mind. Don't measure what you did against anyone else, or even against your ultimate goal. If you moved more today than yesterday, you're improving already! Now focus on what you can do tomorrow.

If you have trouble exercising because your physical condition is too deteriorated, then follow the developmental stages you went through to develop your bones in the first place. Get yourself into water; start with moving in a warm bath, if necessary, and when you can do that, proceed to a warm hot tub or pool. Next add weight resistance in the water. From there you'll eventually progress to being able to return to strenuous movement on land. You'll be moving back up the phyologenetic scale, from jellyfish to human!

Keep in mind that swimming, although it is a good place to start, has less benefit for bones than weight bearing activities. So, as soon as you can do so safely, include some walking. Later, you can add biking, or even jogging or aerobics. Playing tennis, basketball, jumping on a trampoline, jumping rope and weight lifting are beneficial too.

The key to reaping the benefits of exercise is to build it into your daily routine and to have fun. So, if you use an appointment book or calendar, make an appointment with yourself, and then exercise during that time. If that's too big a step, then use that appointment time to shape a plan and decide what's possible.

Since it's easy to exercise the jaw muscle, you could even begin by talking with someone about your exercise goals and ask for their ideas and support. Start by checking in with your health care provider to help you assess where your fitness level is now and to find out what a realistic beginning step might be for you. Then talk to a staff member at a health and fitness club whose job it is to help people assess what they need and begin. If talking is your favorite activity, then combine a fitness activity with visits with friends. Take a walk, swim, or visit a health or fitness club together.

Some people keep their bones strong because their job involves physical labor. If your job is sedentary, consider a hobby that involves physical work, like gardening, or taking care of horses, for example. That will make it easy for you to stay motivated. You don't have to spend money on a hobby or a health club, however. Walking is the easiest weight-bearing exercise; it costs nothing, requires no special equipment and provides marvelous benefits for bones.

How Often? Once you have your bone-building activities decided, how often do you need to do them for maximum bone bank benefit? For aerobic, weight-bearing activity, most sources recommend a minimum of three 20–30 minute sessions per week. For strength training, dietician Sharon Bortz, M.S., R.D., reports excellent effects from strength training only two days a week. In a study she worked on at the Human Nutrition Research Center on Aging at Tufts University in Boston, "The women started with a 5-minute warm-up of light aerobic activity... then performed two sets of eight repetitions. The resistance was set at levels that did not allow them to do more than eight reps. Once they could do more, the resistance was increased." The study emphasized working the muscles "most used for activities of daily living; namely the knee extension, double leg press, lateral pulldown, back extension, and the abdominal curl." Apparently these activities work because "muscle mass is directly related to strength and strength is related to bone mass."[8]

Such aerobic, weight-bearing activities and resistance exercises also have been shown to build bone mass in men. "Men who reported regular exercise had significantly higher BMD (bone mineral density) at the spine and hip."[9]

Whether your activity is aerobic or resistance exercise, include some stretches in your routine. Always stretch after your muscles are warmed up, not before. And remember, your body needs time to build up. Slow and steady wins the race. One physician tells his patients that "It takes time for this process to occur, therefore you don't want to increase stresses too fast—that will make a stress fracture. Therefore, build up slowly when exercising."[10]

However, too much of a good thing is no longer a good thing, so don't overdo it! Bad bones can happen to good people when they get more exercise than their hormonal systems can handle. Reducing body fat too low results in low hormone production, and these are key factors in the setup for osteoporosis! Studies show that problems with bone loss develop when levels of physical activity are so high that they are associated with impaired ovulation.[11] If you try to make exercise the only part of what you do to prevent osteoporosis, you could be very sorry.

Carol Gieg (whom we met in Chapters 1 and 2) exercised constantly from childhood on. She walked, she hiked, biked, went kayaking, and so forth. If exercise were the only answer to bone health, she should have had fabulous, perfect bones. Instead, she has had numerous stress fractures and severe osteoporosis, as demonstrated in bone density measurements. Her predicament is a good reminder that exercise is not the only answer to perfect bones. It is one part of the answer. Exercise must be balanced with proper nutrition designed for your particular body's needs.

As Mary Jane Mack, R.N., points out, "When bodies are deficient in the first place, exercise will be hard and people won't get to peak performance. They feel tired. People may drive themselves, but underneath they're still deficient in nutrients, which means they lack the nutritional foundation to fuel the process. Exercising alone cannot correct the deficiency, and may do more harm. One example is when people's heart electricity is low and they drive themselves to exercise. If their main battery [their heart] is weak, then the whole system will weaken. After short or long term, their body can't handle it and they wind up with more chronic problems . . . including stress fractures or more serious types of fractures, among other things."[12]

That's why Bruce West, D.C., puts people who need to rebuild their bones on concentrated nutritional protocols for 30 to 60 days before recommending they start exercising, and then insists they have a trainer. "They are in a real catch 22. Most are in relatively severe pain which makes them immobile, but they need to be active to recover. That's why they have to have a trainer. Almost anyone can develop a weight bearing program, paraplegics, anybody. It may seem like a minor amount of weight, but even a tiny amount of weight will help."

Metabolic Activity

Physical activity speeds up metabolic activity, the rate at which the body breaks down and uses food. Therefore good digestive activity and absorption of foods is central to the good blood quality upon which bones depend. As Michael Dobbins, D.C., points out, "We are what we eat, based on what we metabolize."[13] In other words, truly to improve our nutritional state, we must not only eat well, but metabolize well.

Digestive Movement. The materials in food become bone through being processed and absorbed in different "rooms" of the digestive system. Although located inside the body, this system is actually a continuation of the *outside* of the body! Its mucous lining (mucosa) and cells are an extension of the skin. The digestive lining helps keep the outside out; if that protective lining breaks down, unwanted particles can get through into the body. The digestive lining is not only the first line of absorption, it's also the first line of defense.

When digestion doesn't work properly, bones never receive the deposits they need. The sometimes noisy and obvious symptoms of digestive problems can be a first indication that bone health is silently declining. Such symptoms often include, among others: bloating, belching, gas, diarrhea or constipation, stomach or intestinal pain, food allergies, rectal itching, and acne.

Digestive insufficiencies are also associated with certain diseases. According to the American Council on Collaborative Medicine, they include: Addison's disease, asthma, celiac disease, dermatitis herpetiformis, diabetes mellitus, chronic hives and excema, gallbladder disease, chronic autoimmune disorders, hepatitis, lupus erythematosus, myasthenia gravis, osteoporosis, pernicious anemia, psoriasis, rheumatoid arthritis, rosacea, Sjogren's syndrome, thyrotoxicosis, hyper-and hypothyroidism, and vitiligo.[14]

There are four main "rooms" in which are carried out the activities that keep bones healthy: the mouth, the stomach, the small intestine, and the large intestine.

Mouth. The mouth serves as a reception room for materials destined for the bone bank. It is here that foods are received, "registered" and begin their conversion into healthy bone bank deposits. Two events take place to initiate this modification process. The first is mechanical: the act of chewing. The second is the release of the enzyme ptyalin by the "spit glands" (also called salivary or parotid glands).

Mixing food with ptyalin in the chewing process is the first line of defense within the digestive system because this secretion contains some immune cells (immunoglobulins) that can begin to neutralize anything that could ultimately harm bones. Ptyalin also begins breaking down carbohydrates into a form the stomach can receive (maltose and dextrin). Thus, lack of sufficient chewing or lack of sufficient ptyalin mixed with food renders it unavailable to the rest of the metabolic cycle and ultimately to the bones. But whether sufficiently chewed or not, once swallowed, food descends to the next digestive "room", the stomach.

Stomach. In the second processing room, future bone bank deposits mix with gastric juices containing various enzymes that further break them down. Sufficient hydrochloric acid (HCl) in the stomach is an absolute precondition for absorbing the nutrients bones need. In fact, the calcium bones require can only be absorbed in a sufficiently acidic stomach environment.

That's why it's self-defeating to take a calcium-based antacid and expect bones to benefit from the calcium content. Such antacids result in the stomach having too little acid to complete its tasks. The body has to contend somehow with the unmetabolized calcium, and often deposits it in the wrong places. That's one way calcium ends up in soft tissues. In artery walls it can cause atherosclerosis (hardening of the arteries). In the gallbladder it becomes gall stones. In the kidney, it forms kidney stones. If deposited in the ear drum, it can harden the filmy eardrum and prevents it from vibrating, thus contributing to deafness.

Indeed, C.R.A.™ practitioner Mary Jane Mack, R.N., says the most common digestive problem that contributes to poor bone health is "lack of hydrochloric acid." That's why she checks every person to see if they're able to absorb bone nutrients. If not, she adds Zypan (SP) or Betaine (SP) to their protocols (see below). She adds that some people are unable to take either one because the mucosal lining of their stomach is so thin they can't handle taking this nutrition. In that case, she recommends Okra Pepsin (SP). Sometimes, depending on how much healing the stomach needs, she's had to "start people very slowly to get them absorbing nutrition before even starting to deliver the other nutrients they need." This circumstance, she points out, is most common in people whose "blood quality is very low, so low they can't even handle the nutrition. In turn, the most common causes of that are parasites or chemicals in the system that deplete the blood" (see Chapter 11).[15]

Low levels of the mineral zinc are another factor when foods are not properly metabolized (see also Part Two, Chapters 6 and 7). This is especially likely when when someone experiences many food cravings. States Dr. Versendaal, "The body is craving the cofactors that make the stomach work, and one of the main cofactors is often zinc." In his experience, the more overweight a person is, and the more they crave, the more zinc they are likely to need. "Without zinc", he adds, "nothing can work in the body."

That's because zinc is an essential component of all the bodily tissues that develop from the ectoderm—the outer layer of cells in a developing embryo. These include all the skin structures, of which the entire gut is one, the nervous system, organs of special sense, the pineal and part of the pituitary and suprarenal glands.

Michael Dobbins, D.C., points to stomach ulcers as another disturbance that can contribute to poor bone health. "Stomach ulcers are bacterial invasions primarily due to lowered resistance due to vitamin deficiencies."[16] Since vitamins carry essential minerals into the bone bank, restoring healthy vitamin levels is a digestive key to perfect bones. Dr. Mack concludes, "Usually if you correct digestion in the stomach, you don't have to correct it below."[17]

Small Intestine/Duodenum. This is the third chamber for processing bone bank deposits. It is where foods are further digested and then absorbed into the bloodstream so they can be carried to the bone bank. For most nutrients, this is both their only and last chance to be absorbed.

To carry out its job, the small intestine receives some help. If dealing with carbohydrates, the pancreas sends assistance. If fats are present, the gallbladder helps out with bile (see Part Two, Chapter 8). If fats cannot be completely processed, there are several negative consequences for the bone bank. One is that the vitamins that fats are supposed to carry to bones cannot be absorbed, resulting in a deficiency of vitamins A, D, E and K, despite adequate amounts in the diet. Another is that unmetabolized fats cannot provide courier service for minerals (see Part Two, Chapter 7).

Still another difficulty for bones can arise from incomplete protein breakdown, an activity carried out in this third digestive space. When proteins are incompletely digested, they cannot carry out their function of building the connective tissue mesh that receives bone bank deposits, thus weakening the connective tissue and ultimately, the bones (see Part Two, Chapter 6).

Digestive processes in the intestine are greatly aided by friendly flora—intestinal bacteria. Without their help, digestion cannot be completed. That's a problem many people encounter as a result of taking antibiotics. These drugs destroy friendly intestinal flora along with disease-causing bacteria. Again, digestion remains incomplete, and bone building nutrients cannot arrive at the bone bank. Also, without friendly intestinal bacteria, the stage is set for an overgrowth of undesirable microbes such as yeast (Candida) which embezzle bone nutrients and spend their riches on themselves (see Part Two, Chapter 11).

The relative health of the mucous membrane of the small intestine has everything to do with whether bones will get what they need. For example, sometimes this membrane becomes damaged, and can leak. Usually, states Dr. Dobbins, this problem starts with an endocrine imbalance, which can result from a lack of the essential fatty acids that keep the mucous membrane healthy. That's why practitioners sometimes recommend Pituitary PMG (see Part Two, Chapter 9) for digestive system support: it is likely to help stimulate ulcers to heal.

The lining of the small intestine can, over time, become coated with a kind of internal sludge. This substance builds up in the same way as creosote in fireplace chimneys. The tar-like substance coats the intestinal walls and prevents nutrients from being absorbed. This is especially likely for people whose intake of refined carbohydrates and sugars has been high. This unwelcome coating can be slowly removed by eating more dietary fiber.

Large Intestines. The last room in the intestines acts as an exit station. The large intestine receives undigested remains of food from the small intestine. Rather than continuing to digest them, the large intestine moves them along (via peristalsis), removes water and, with the help of friendly bacteria, further degrades them in preparation for elimination. Without this job taking place, undigested materials would back up in the system, contaminating and ultimately shutting down the metabolic processes that deliver bone bank nutrients.

Kidneys. The kidneys also contribute to healthy bones. They filter blood, remove other waste products, particularly the minerals sodium and potassium, and retain blood cells, proteins, and other necessary substances. Before eliminating what they have filtered, the kidneys provide one last service to the bone bank: they can selectively reabsorb the minerals calcium, magnesium and potassium that had been destined for elimination, thus giving the bone bank a second chance to deposit them. The kidneys' ability to filter is dependent to a great extent on blood pressure, which is why it's so important to keep blood pressure in the normal range (around 120/80).

The kidneys also play a central role in maintaining proper pH balance. Without their constant vigilance in adjusting acid-base ratios, the nutrients bones need could not be absorbed (see Part Two, Chapter 7). As Dr. Dobbins points out, "When there's a pH imbalance, it's always a kidney problem."[18]

Activities Done to Bones

Both the voluntary movements of exercise and the passive movements of the metabolic cycle are affected by one last bodily activity: the movement of nerve impulses. If these impulses become blocked, the organs and muscles for which they were destined will never receive them. Without a free flow of nerve messages, the function of these organs and muscles will be inhibited. In turn, messages returning from these organs to the glands and areas of the brain that control them will not be delivered. The proper functioning of these nerve impulses is the foundation of chiropractic practice. Since nutritional imbalances and deficiencies are often at the root of recurrent subluxations, many chiropractors include nutritional work as part of their practice.[19]

Because nerve impulses travel through the spine and near and around various other bones and joints, chiropractors adjust these bones to align them one to another, to free up nerves that might be "pinched" and therefore not able to send their crucial messages all the way to their destinations. When bones are out of alignment, they can cause difficulties with proper absorption. Whether misalignments are in the spine, the wrists, shoulders, or ankles, it is important to bring them back into alignment. However, a sudden adjustment can snap the bones of someone with severe osteoporosis. Therefore, in case your body worker is unaware of the state of your bone health, take care of yourself by informing him or her, and refuse methods of adjustment that require sudden thrusts. There are other, gentle and equally effective ways to produce good alignment.

If your health care practitioner is a chiropractor, it is likely he or she will check your alignment and make necessary corrections. For example, Dr. Versendaal reports, he or she "may need to adjust the right carpal bone to kick start the hormonal system." Other adjustments particularly important in bone health include: the 4th and 5th cervical vertebrae, both thumbs, the right ring finger, and the carpal (wrist) bones. These areas, among other things, control circuits relating to the parathyroid gland, the uterus and prostate, the liver, and various other hormone factories.[20]

If your practitioner knows C.R.A.™ and is not a chiropractor, he or she can test you to find out if something's out of place, and then refer you to a chiropractor for further care.

In addition to chiropractic, there is a gentle method of body-work that provides direct stimulation to bones. Called *Zero Balancing*, and presented in the book of the same name authored by Fritz Smith, M.D., it is both subtle and powerful. A trained practitioner can stimulate bones by applying slight pressure and movement to the muscles that attach to the bones.

Finally, since proper alignment is central to bone health, foot orthotics may be necessary to provide crucial support to the body framework and organ systems. Some health professionals are able to test for whether or not orthotics are indicated.

Protocols

MOUTH:

Parotid (SP) contains nutritional support for the parotid gland. It may be recommended to help rid the body of environmental toxins such as those from mercury amalgam dental fillings or from viruses that attack the parotid gland, such as mumps. It's also recommended in chemical poisoning, for people who've been on chemotherapy or those who are exposed to valley fever. Dr. Michael Dobbins reports it's also excellent for people with silver amalgam fillings that are leaking, even if they don't get the tooth fixed."[21] It is also designed to support the relationship between the salivary glands (parotids) and thyroid. Practitioners often recommend 6 Parotid PMG for 12 weeks.

Paraplex (SP) provides nutritional support for use when low parotid (salivary gland) output is secondary to hormonal imbalances, especially in the pituitary, thyroid, pancreas, and adrenal glands. Practitioners may recommend 3–6 a day.

STOMACH:

Okra Pepsin E3 (SP) provides nutritional support to help break down mucous when there's so much covering the intestinal wall that food can't be readily absorbed into the blood. Okra is sticky and adheres to the intestinal wall long enough to put the protein digesting enzyme, pepsin, in contact with the protein-based mucous. It's especially helpful in colitis, diverticulitis, ulcers, malabsorption syndrome, and ileocecal valve problems.

Dr. Michael Dobbins adds, it "has the factors found in cabbage juice that have such healing powers. Therefore it has a role in addressing diarrhea, constipation, indigestion, intestinal flu, colitis, and gouty diathesis. It also contains vitamin E factors and other agents that support tissue repair."[22] He recommends taking it on an empty stomach, so it can coat the stomach directly, without interference from food. Practitioners usually recommend 6 a day, but in acute cases, they may recommend 9.[23]

Zypan (SP) aids the digestive process of the stomach by helping to normalize its acidity, which should be highly acid, at a pH of 2 or 3. It is therefore central to the absorption of calcium and iron. It also helps the stomach digest carbohydrates, fats, and proteins. When practitioners recommend it to address nutritional needs for stomach digestion, they may use 6–15 a day. When they suggest it to assist absorption of other protocols, the recommended amount may be less.

Betaine (SP) is designed to make hydrochloric acid available to the stomach, which aids in the digestion of protein and minerals. It's often recommended in a dosage of 3–6 a day for people suffering from gas, indigestion, malassimilation, demineralization and pernicious anemia.

Gastrex (SP) contains okra powder, discussed above, and bentonite (nutritional clay). It is often recommended to immediately relieve an over-acid stomach. The function of the clay is to draw toxins to itself for removal. Gastrex also contains tillandsia, which lubricates, adsorbs and helps eliminate. Together, the combination helps "put out the fire" (inflammation), eliminate toxins, and provide a mucous membrane healing agent, Okra Pepsin. Practitioners often recommend 2 about 10 minutes before eating.

Zinc-Liver Chelate provides the zinc necessary to activate the digestive processes. Because zinc feeds all the organs that arise from the ectoderm (listed above), it is useful for digestive insufficiencies, nervous system disorders, immune insufficiency, slow rates of healing, reduced sex drive, prostatic hypertrophy, loss of sense of smell and/or taste, chronic yeast infections, failing eye sight, hair loss, gray hair. It is also necessary that zinc be present in order to make vitamin D work. One indication of zinc deficiency is white spots on the fingernails. Some practitioners use it for short-term zinc needs (less than 2 months), and, for longer term, use Chezyn (see below), which contains a balanced ratio of zinc, copper and iron. Others recommend zinc-liver chelate long-term but not Chezyn. However it is used, Zinc needs to be balanced with copper for optimum body functioning.

SMALL INTESTINE:

Betafood and AF Betafood (SP) to support the gallbladder and breakdown of oils, were covered in Chapter 8, Dry Bones and Essential Fatty Acids.

Cataplex GTF (SP) contains food factors that help increase insulin production in the pancreas and the cells' response to insulin. It is often recommended for nutritional support for low blood sugar (hypoglycemia), high blood sugar (hyperglycemia) or insulin production problems. It may also be used for its anti-arteriosclerosis function, as research points to its presence retarding the formation of arterial plaques of cholesterol and calcium that can adhere to the blood vessel walls.

Chezyn (SP) was addressed in Chapter 7, Making Abundant Deposits.

LARGE INTESTINE:

Spanish Black Radish (SP): See Chapter 11.

KIDNEYS:

Albaplex (SP): See Chapter 11.
A C Carbamide (SP) contains a variety of nutritional factors that support the transfer of body fluids through cell walls. (That process is called osmosis; it allows for elements dissolved in

liquid solution to pass through cell membranes.) Osmosis enables these elements to be used for cell metabolism or to carry out products of elimination. It may be recommended for someone who is retaining water, has swollen extremities, sweat gland symptoms, or kidney and bladder symptoms, including when these health problems stimulate nightmares. (See also Chapter 9.)

Vegetarian protocols are listed below. All products have been described in other chapters.

Mouth: (Parotid Reflex) 3 CalSol, 3 Choline, 3 Spanish Black Radish and 3–6 Zymex II.

Stomach: 3 Black Currant Seed Oil, 3 Chlorophyll Complex, 3 FenGre.

Gut: Zymex II, up to 2 every two hours.

Gallbladder: 6 Betafood, sometimes with the addition of 6 Choline, and/or 3–6 Betaine Hydrochloride.

Duodenum/Small Intestine: 6 Linum B6, 3 FenGre, 3 Lact-Enz.

Pancreas: 6-10 Inositol, 3 Lact-Enz, 6 Betafood and 2 Spanish Black Radish.

Kidneys: 6 A C Carbamide, 3 Spanish Black Radish, 6 Zymex, 1 Organic Iodine.

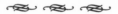

Becoming physically active, supporting the digestive process, and freeing up nerve impulse transmissions through proper alignment can make all the difference in the quest for healthy bones.

But there is one last factor to address. The bone bank must have protection from embezzlers, the subject of Chapter 11.

ENDNOTES

1. *NIH Consensus Statement,* National Institutes of Health, Office of the Director, Volume 12, Number 4, June 6–8, 1994, p. 14.

2. Dover, Ibid., p. 18.
3. Dover, Ibid., p. 18.
4. "Calcium, Beneficial to Bones and More" in *Healthy Cell News*, Spring/Summer 1996, p. 17.
5. *Osteoporosis and You*, Colorado Department of Health, Osteoporosis Prevention Project, PPD-IP-A5, Denver, Colorado, Vol. 1, No. 3.
6. Dover, Ibid., p. 16.
7. Claire Martin. "A Positive Impact," Outside, December 1997, p. 150.
8. Sharon Bortz. "Calcium, Part 3" in *Redwood Health Club Newsletter*, November 1997, p. 1.
9. E. J. Bendavid, J. Shan, and E. Barrett-Conner. "Factors Associated with Bone Mineral Density in Middle-Aged Men." *Journal of Bone Mineral Res.* 11, no. 8 (August 1996): 1185–90.
10. Available at: http://www.os2bbs.com/malka/osteopRX.htm
11. Gaby, Ibid., p. 147.
12. Mack, Author's Interview, Ibid.
13. Dobbins, Ibid.
14. *American Council on Collaborative Medicine*, Vol. IV, Issue 5, May 1998.
15. Mack, Author's Interview, Ibid.
16. Dobbins, Ibid.
17. Mack, Author's Interview, Ibid.
18. Dobbins, Ibid.
19. Fred Ulan, D.C., C.C.N., "Preventing Recurring Subluxations with CRA" in *The American Chiropractor*, Sept./Oct. 1998, pp. 26–40.
20. D. A. Versendaal, D.C., Ph.D., "Brittle Bone Syndrome," C.R.A.™ Seminar Educational Materials, p. 2.
21. Dobbins, Ibid.
22. Dobbins, Ibid.
23. Dobbins, Ibid.

CHAPTER ELEVEN

Strengthening Security Systems: Protecting Bones from Robbers, Embezzlers and Bone Leachers

Wherever there are riches, there are likely to be attempts to access them by those for whom they were not intended. The mineral treasures meant for bones are certainly no exception. Robbers, embezzlers, and bone leachers stand ready to remove hard-won bone bank deposits during any lapse in security. Thus, the final component of the Six-Point Plan for Perfect Bones addresses how to sustain sufficient protection to keep bones' treasure secure.

Bones have always needed protection. However, safeguarding them in the modern world is more important than it has ever been. Air pollution, for example, adversely impacts 4 to 5 billion people worldwide. Mary Jane Mack, R.N., explains the connection to bone health: "More people are deficient [in bone-building nutrients] today because of indoor and outdoor pollution. The houses are so well insulated they don't breathe. The house has no filter system, so pollution builds up in the house. Many chemicals are used in cleaning, new products in houses, weed and feed chemicals around the houses, chemical lawns. These are all toxins that deplete the blood. People feel sick after they spray their yard, then they go to a resort to get better, but that place is sprayed with chemicals inside and out.

"And then there's radiation in the air from computers, cell phones, pagers. These emissions deplete the blood, the vitamins and iron, because the body can't handle it, it's like a foreign substance. These pollutants are at such levels today that the average person has a hard time keeping above it. If your body's a little unhealthy in the first place, you don't have a chance. Osteoporosis is the end result. The most common cause is the outdoor pollution. Women have achy bones, because their bones swell, they'll complain of joint or bone aches. I'm seeing it more in men now too."[1]

Sources suggest that "Americans are threatened daily by over 100,000 different synthetic chemicals. Shockingly, there are over one-half trillion pounds in the United States alone!"[2] And, an estimated 1,000 new ones are introduced every year, only a couple hundred of which have been tested for health effects. And of those which have been tested, few have been checked for health effects in children and developing infants.[3] This fact alone means the bone health of the new generation may already be severely impacted, long before they reach what are considered to be the "at risk" years for declining bone health.

In fact, the U.S. government is stepping up research on many of these chemicals because they may be "hormone disrupting", the signs of which are unnaturally early puberty for girls, lower sperm counts in men, increased rates of cancer, sterility and developmental problems.[4]

It all adds up to the need for a strong, effective security system to protect bone bank deposits. Maintaining a security system that is truly effective requires some knowledge of the modus operandi of the various and nefarious culprits. Knowing how they work provides answers for how to prevent them from making a getaway with bones' treasures. And, astonishing as it may seem, the bone-robber most frequently encountered wears a friendly, familiar face: that of the food that comprises the modern diet.

Food

Few people would consciously decide to give up long-term bone health by inviting known bone-robbers to take up bodily residence. Yet that is exactly what happens on a daily basis when we consume many modern "foods". To comprehend the modern foodstuffs' role in damaging bones is to step behind the scenes of present-day food production and be confronted with processes that could confound a rocket scientist.

The story begins with seeds (many now genetically altered) which are grown on depleted soil that is soaked with chemical fertilizers. This "food" is then sprayed with pesticides during its growth. (For a thorough treatment of this subject, see Jensen and Anderson's *Empty Harvest*.)

From there, reports Alan Gaby, M.D., modern food is then "bleached, radiated, extracted with organic solvents, subjected to enormous temperatures and extremes of acidity or alkalinity and contaminated with thousands of chemicals designed to preserve, texturize, color, or otherwise modify the food so that it will look, feel, and taste like the real thing."[5]

The results of these processes are foods that look like foods, but act in the body as what nutritionist Bob LeRoy, R.D., labels "calcium antagonists", and what Dr. Versendaal calls "counterfeit". However they are labeled, the more we consume such processed "food", the more negative are the ramifications for bone health.

Mary Jane Mack, R.N., explains that such processed foods are electrically negative (levo-rotatory), while those that promote bone health (and overall health) are electrically positive (dextro-rotatory). C.R.A.™ practitioners can actually test the electrical charge of a food in the same way they can test the charge of a body reflex. "If an orange or an apple is really healthy, new, organic, it's more likely to test positive."[6] Fortunately, one need not become a C.R.A.™ practitioner to know which foods are positive, and which negative. In general, live, fresh, whole foods are positively charged, while processed, chemically preserved, highly sugared foods or old and stale ones are negatively charged.

She adds, "Positive foods spin to the right, and they build the body up at a cellular level; they give the person more energy and make the body healthier. Anything negatively charged pulls the health of the body down; it moves through the body slowly, therefore causing debris, which can even cause stones. Negatively charged food causes buildup in the liver and gallbladder: sludge. A lot of synthetic vitamins are negatively charged."[7]

Electrically negative foods, says Dr. Versendaal, cause the human body to make dangerous substitutions in its structure. The body takes in and uses these counterfeit and imitation foods and chemicals "in an attempt to compensate for the lack of natural elements." Microbes, he adds, eagerly pounce on bodies so constructed as soon as the slightest breakdown in security occurs.[8]

The fact that such foods both substitute chemicals for real mineral treasure and lower the effectiveness of the bone bank's security system are two reasons nutritionist Bob LeRoy, R.D., defines such negatively charged food as part of a "calcium-draining lifestyle": "Evidence is mounting...that osteoporosis is not a disease of calcium deficiency, but rather the result of lifestyle choices that speed up calcium excretion from the bones. Consuming massive doses of calcium, whether through falsely-reassuring dairy products or mega-supplements, cannot be expected to counteract a 'calcium-draining' lifestyle."

He insists that we need to reduce, and in some cases avoid, the 'calcium antagonists' over which we have control. These include "above all others, animal protein and excess total protein; importantly, sedentary habits; and, to varying degrees, sodium chloride, smoking, vitamin D overdosing or sunlight deprivation, caffeine, steroids, alcoholism, aluminum, fluorides, refined sweeteners, and serious calcium/magnesium or calcium/phosphorus dietary imbalances."[9] (See Chapter 11 for a discussion of these bone leachers and embezzlers, along with protocols to address them.)

Other experts concur. In fact, the National Institutes of Health issued a statement summarizing the present knowledge of these authorities. Their consensus was that "urinary loss accounts for approximately 50 percent [of calcium loss]. The typical American diet consists of high amounts of sodium and animal protein, both of which can significantly increase urinary calcium excretion."[10]

Additionally, even food that was healthy to begin with, when undigested, can turn to poison in the body, attacking the very systems it was consumed to support.[11] This is how digestive problems contribute to a "calcium-draining" lifestyle. One factor that can lead to food remaining unassimilated is a pH imbalance. States Dr. Versendaal, "I believe that the body should be slightly acid: 6.3 to 6.5, in that area, as measured by a litmus test on the tongue. If it's off, you can't heal. As soon as the stomach pH goes from acid to alkaline, that means the stomach's ability to produce enzymes and hydrochloric acid is shut down. The body overnight becomes alkaline and the body poisons itself. The food is not digested and becomes rotten and putrefies. It literally attacks and weakens the body."

He adds, "If you take too much food, it can be bad for you. The old saying is, "One apple is good for you, two apples give you gas, and three apples will give you diarrhea." You're changing your pH. Apples will make you highly alkaline if you eat too many of them. Then your body becomes toxic, tired, weak, run down. It's like if you never went to bed for a week—your body would become toxic from not sleeping and recouping. A lot of people get alkaline bodies from sleep deprivation."[12]

Food allergies may also contribute to poor bone health. Since foods to which one is allergic are incompletely digested, they change pH and reduce absorption of essential nutrients. To find out what food intolerances people have, practitioners may recommend an elimination diet: removing a suspected food from the diet for a period of time and then adding it again to see if it causes a reaction. Another way is to eliminate the foods known to be hard for one's blood type to tolerate. (See the lists in Peter D'Adamo's *Eat Right for Your Type*.)

High on the inventory of negatively charged "foods" and also the list of "foods" having a profound negative effect on bone health are refined carbohydrates and sugar. Because they contain few or no vitamins or minerals themselves, in order to be metabolized these "foods" use the riches meant for the bone bank. In other words, these foods rob the bone bank of its mineral deposits. Additionally, sugar actually *causes* the body to release calcium. "Since 99% of the total-body calcium is in our bones, this increase in calcium excretion most likely reflects a leaching of calcium from bone."[13] Nutritionist Royal Lee, D.D.S., stated that glucose (the most common sugar we consume) blocks the assimilation of calcium.[14]

Dr. Versendaal paints a graphic portrait of this process, "Sugar will leach bones, and everybody eats sugar. Sugar is electrically negative, it destroys blood, it destroys teeth. If you talk to a dentist and say what's the one thing you could eat or drink that destroys teeth, they'll say sugar. Teeth are nothing but bone. Sugar burns up the bone marrow, it eats up bone. The way sugar is made, it's bleached and no longer natural, it erodes bone, takes its minerals. The body tries to fight back, but what bone is left is going to erode, collapse, deteriorate."

A recent study by researchers at the U.S. Department of Agriculture reported that "drinking lots of non-diet soft drinks can weaken your bones... the fructose sweetener in the [non-diet] drinks led to severe losses of bone-building phosphorous and calcium," a situation worsened fivefold in people with low magnesium intake.[15]

One form of sugar that is particularly harmful to bones is corn syrup, which is added to breakfast cereals, fruit drinks and a host of other foods. States Bruce West, D.C., "It is the only sugar that causes diabetes in test animals because it destroys the pancreas' insulin producing cells. It also blocks the assimilation of calcium in your body. And the end result can be osteoporosis and arthritis, two other epidemic diseases in this country."[16]

Does that mean consuming absolutely no sugar? Mary Jane Mack, R.N., answers that if sugar "is just one ingredient I don't worry about it. When someone is in a critical state, though, they have a hard time managing sugar. They don't realize until they get off of it, how tired they were from trying to handle the sugar. Taking a lot of sugar daily depletes the nutrition in the body and weakens their system and opens it for breakdown, including osteoporosis."[17] To give the body the real nutrient it needs when it signals a sugar craving, she recommends taking inositol, one of the B vitamins (see below).

Similar to sugar in its bone-robbing effect is alcohol. People who drink excessively risk osteoporosis, partly due to the deficient diet that usually accompanies drinking, and partly to the toxicity of the alcohol. Alcohol dissolves and depletes the vitamin B complex, among other things. It is toxic to the liver and it dissolves the crystalline mineral deposits that have been held in the bone bank. As Michael Dobbins, D.C., points out, "Excessive alcohol ingestion destroys liver cells, which results in a massive tissue antibody response. In a normal person this will normalize itself. The body produces histamine (in response to ingested toxins) which increases tissue permeability to help clean out. Anti-histamines [either produced by the body or ingested] stop the histamine reaction. If the person stops ingesting alcohol soon enough, the liver will self-repair in a short time provided that the person is otherwise healthy."

Caffeine is another bone leacher. It causes the body to excrete calcium at a rapid rate. Routinely ingesting a lot of caffeine, either in colas, coffee, or strong black teas, forces the bone bank into a deficit spending mode.

Smoking tobacco also has a direct negative effect on bones, although the reasons for this are not completely understood. The nicotine in tobacco is closely related chemically to the nutrient niacinamide. Inhaling tobacco causes nicotine to take up residence where the nutrient niacinamide belongs. One of the key places is in the nerves. Smoking nicotine is addictive in part because it throws the body deeper and deeper into a niacinamide deficit, which accounts for the frayed nerves of a smoker craving a cigarette. Part of smoking's negative effect on bones is presumed to be from toxins or chemicals in the smoke (see the metal cadmium, below).

Does this mean that to keep the bone bank secure, we have to stay rigidly away from all such negatively charged foods and substances? No, says Michael Dobbins, D.C. He points out that even "Royal Lee said, in a well-fed individual, the body can deal with a little smoking and drinking. It's not the tobacco or alcohol [or sugar or caffeine] alone, it's the [combination of these toxins with] the debilitated state, and now the denatured food."[18]

Synthetic Chemicals

Maureen Schaub, whose hormonal imbalances contributed to bone loss, as described in Chapter 9, found out that her occupation constantly exposed her to bone-robbing toxic chemicals. As a beautician, she was constantly breathing them in from hair dyes, perms and other chemical agents. Even though she had significant hormonal imbalances, her body needed to deal with chemical poisoning as the first priority in regaining her bone health. Because she is still constantly exposed at work, she continues to take a small amount of Parotid (SP) daily, a product designed to clean chemical poisons from the body.

For Sophia Tampinelli, whose many layers of healing were described in Part One, Chapter 5, dealing with chemical poisoning was also the first layer on the road back to bone health. However, she is unaware of the source of these toxins. What she does know is that when she attended a seminar with Dr. Versendaal, "He said I had an enlarged heart and a fallen or collapsed body due to chemical poisoning." Like Maureen, she also took Parotid. Although Dr. Versendaal also found hormonal imbalances at the time, he was concerned that Sophia's heart was too weak to handle the fluids she'd likely start to eliminate once she began her second layer of healing, sex hormone support. Therefore he advised her to wait to take this second protocol until after the Parotid protocol. That way her heart would be strong enough to successfully pump out the massive release of fluids which would occur in her second layer of healing. Indeed, this proved to be true. She lost 24 pounds of fluids in the first few months.

Dr. Versendaal was not surprised that Sophia was unaware of the source of her chemical poisoning. He recounts, "In recent years over 60,000 synthetic chemicals have been added to our world. The oceans and waterways are so polluted that any of the life-forms that live in and drink from it are victims of [early] sickness, aging, and death. The air is poison—the earth is drenched with chemical fertilizers, pesticides and chemicals...We consume toxic chemistry in virtually every type of food or drink we purchase. Synthetic poisons and chemicals have permeated our homes and work places...in carpets, paints, and cosmetics. The drinking water that pours out of our taps is filled with chemicals, heavy metals, and toxins that make us frail. The widespread use of antibiotics has created powerful strains of mutant bacteria and fungi."[19]

Certainly one important source of chemical poisoning is prescription drugs. Although usually thought of as substances that support health, drugs prescribed for an apparently unrelated symptom can rob bones directly, or else compromise the bone bank security system, leaving bones susceptible to being plundered. For example, as pointed out in Chapter 9, keeping hormone "factories" in good production is central to bone health. But Dan Newell, N.C., explains that drugs can cause "a shift in endocrine compensation. For example, someone who has been hypothyroid may have developed such a chloride-sodium shift which has created such a pH imbalance that that's what you're fighting primarily…which the drugs can cause."

One circumstance in which drugs promote bone loss is taking standard pharmaceuticals for thyroid problems and for estrogen replacement at the same time. Estrogen will block the effect of the thyroid medication, reports John Lee, M.D. However, natural progesterone enhances utilization of thyroid hormone.[20]

The class of drugs called antibiotics can promote bone burglaries indirectly. Dr. Dobbins explains that's because antibiotics suppress the immune system's signals to spring into action.[21] While the security system's capacity to respond is diminished, antibiotics inadvertently make the bone bank accessible to be burglarized.

A partial list of other prescription drugs that have a bone robbing effect can be found in Part One, Chapter 3, under treatments that damage bones. The more such drugs are combined, the less anyone, even one's primary physician, can understand their effects. According to Bruce West, D.C., "if just three prescriptions are given, it is now considered a general fact that no doctor or pharmacist can understand the myriad of dangerous interactions between these drugs, your disease, and your body."[22]

Metals

Metals are a class of substances whose members can negatively impact bone deposits. High on the list of such offenders is aluminum, which accumulates in bones, reducing new bone bank deposits, speeding up bone bank withdrawals and stimulating urinary excretion. Aluminum also interferes with the construction of the collagen net that receives deposits, thus it participates in destroying the bank itself![23]

To guard bones against toxic aluminum, it is best to avoid ingesting it by

- consuming juice or soft drinks from glass bottles, not cans or aluminum-lined cartons,
- using only aluminum-free antacids
- using stainless steel or glass cooking utensils,
- filtering drinking and cooking water, or using bottled water from a reputable company,
- avoiding processed foods, as these often contain aluminum, and
- refraining from using underarm deodorants that contain aluminum (usually as aluminum chloride or other salts of aluminum.

Lead is also a bone-robbing culprit. Apparently it displaces calcium in the bone bank, thus increasing the rate of calcium withdrawal. Additionally, it interferes with the hormone progesterone, so necessary for regulating the bone bank. "Unacceptably high levels of lead are found in our air, water, food and soils."[24] Indeed, people with chronic lead poisoning show evidence of osteoporosis. States Alan Gaby, M.D., "We cannot rule out the possibility that a lifetime of low-level lead exposure is one of the factors contributing to the epidemic of osteoporosis in industrialized societies."[25]

Excess exposure to the metal cadmium, especially concentrated in cigarette smoke, contributes to a softening of the bones and resultant fractures.[26]

In sufficient concentrations, tin can reduce calcium content in bones. Tin also inhibits the production of hydrochloric acid in the stomach. Therefore it prevents deposits from ever being processed to arrive in the bone bank.[27] It is present in cans used to store food, toothpastes, some fungicides, insecticides, stabilizers, in packaging materials and in the atmosphere as an industrial pollutant.

Silver amalgam fillings may also contribute to osteoporosis because they can leak the toxic metal mercury. "Mercury is a bioaccumulative neurotoxin linked to damage to the brain, kidneys and fetuses."[28] States Donald Warren, D.D.S., "There always seems to be an increased plaque deposit around mercury amalgam restorations. The plaque toxin and the electrogalvanic current created by that restoration can accelerate bone loss adjacent to the filling."[29] Luckily, "the fresh leaves of cilantro have been shown to mobilize mercury and other toxic metals from the central nervous system if large enough amounts are consumed daily... Dried cilantro does not work."[30]

Infections

A nutritionally deficient body filled with synthetic chemicals and drugs is an environment weakened to the point of being unable to defend itself against disease-causing microorganisms. In turn, these living invaders wreak havoc on the mineral treasure intended for the bone bank. Whether bacterial, viral, parasitic, or yeast, each infectious agent interferes with the metabolic cycle of bone bank deposits and withdrawals in its own unique way. For example, bacteria such as staph (staphylococcus) or strep (streptococcus) not only eat bone, but also secrete toxins that harm bones.

Yeasts, such as Monilia or Candida, can suffocate the oxygen supply needed for bones' metabolic processes. Candida is especially relevant today because of overuse of antibiotics. These kill off the normal flora in the intestines which are part of the security system for the intestinal tract. Without these "healthy bugs", yeasts overgrow, cross through the intestinal membrane and grow throughout the body. Systemically, they use up bone nutrients, including precious oxygen. Additionally, yeast don't help digest food the way their friendly cousins, the intestinal bacteria, do; thus deposits intended for bone never reach the bank.

Viruses rob bones by entering into the cell and taking over the DNA that normally directs cell activities. Therefore viruses affect bones in a variety of ways, depending on the kind of virus and the kind of cells they take over. Viruses can seek out any kind of tissue, and are thus responsible for a wide range of symptoms and illnesses, including smallpox, chickenpox, measles, mumps, the common cold, rabies, epidemic encephalitis, viral pneumonia, AIDS, and long-term chronic conditions such as fibromyalgia.

One way viruses can affect bone health is by attacking connective tissue. This removes the collagen net where bone deposits are made, effectively getting rid of the bone bank itself. Viruses can also attack the nerve supply to bones, or affect the circulation of blood to the bones. Nonetheless, points out Dr. Dobbins, "A virus in an environment that will allow it to replicate will do so, and will not in other environments."[31] Therefore, the key to avoiding such problems is to keep as healthy as possible so as not to provide an environment where viruses can reproduce.

Parasites are yet another form of bone robber. They take the nutrition intended for bones and eat it themselves, thus proliferating themselves while starving their host. Dr. Versendaal reports he finds a lot of parasite problems in California that "show up as itchy skin and teeth grinding," among other things.[32] Parasites are a common finding when testing people whose bone health is deteriorating. These uninvited guests can cause a host of symptoms, many of which may seem unrelated to an infestation, including abdominal pain or cramps, anorexia, autoimmune diseases, chronic fatigue, constipation, diarrhea, distention, fever, food allergies, gastritis, inflammatory bowel disease, low back pain, rash, weight loss, arthritis, colitis, flatulence, headaches, and vomiting, to name a few.

Fungi are vegetable cellular organisms that feed on organic matter such as bacteria and molds. Many are not particularly pathogenic until they encounter a compromised, i.e., poorly nourished or unhealthy host. For that reason, when fungi are present, health professionals suspect serious diseases. Other varieties of fungus that can cause primary infections occur in particular geographic regions such as coccidioidomycoses in the Southwestern U.S., histoplasmosis in the East and Midwest, and paracoccidioidomycoses in South America. Because they feed on organic matter, they can eat the friendly bacteria needed in the G.I. tract, without which the digestive process remains incomplete. They can also enter the system through decayed teeth, which are themselves a sign of compromised bone health.

The key to fighting off all these bone-robbers is a healthy immune system. And, as Dr. Dobbins points out, "the fuel to run the immune system is calcium. The [immune] cells send out little ladders and push during phagocytosis; these are crystalline based and require calcium.

"The immune system is the only thing that can permanently destroy a virus. The immune system has to plug up the holes in the cell that allow those viral pieces through the cell wall and into the cell's DNA...The immune system will plug up the hole in the cell wall with antibodies, which takes time. The viruses will ALWAYS replicate when the environment allows it. The most important factor in this is calcium bicarbonate in the bloodstream and carbamide which maintains the insulating values of the body fluids. In their deficiency, the nucleus and cytoplasm lose their opposite electrical charges, and the cell is dead when the charge is all gone."[33]

One last type of bone leacher is a thoroughly modern invention: nuclear power. During the last decade, Dr. Versendaal has travelled around the United States conducting an average of 3 to 4 days of training sessions per month. Because he has C.R.A.™ tested as many as 150 people at each of these sessions, he has had a unique opportunity to notice patterns of health and illness specific to each locality. He reports that he can always tell when someone lives near a nuclear power plant.

Apparently the good news is that infection rates are lower, he thinks because nuclear energy kills such microorganisms. However, the bad news, he says, is that the oils are all dried up in people's bodies. What that means for bones, as described in Part Two, Chapter 8, is that there are too few carriers to transport minerals to the bone bank, and too few essential fatty acids to make sufficient hormones to regulate the bone bank. (Protocols for correcting these lapses in bone security are also in Chapter 8.)

Before leaving the subject of robbers and embezzlers, a brief discussion of fluoride is warranted. As you may recall from Part One, Chapter 3, fluoride has been put forth as a medical treatment for osteoporosis. Indeed, it helps form bones and teeth, and its administration has been shown to increase bone mineral density test results. However, it also renders these denser bones more brittle. Bone mineral density studies do not measure the suppleness of bone, a factor which is as central to bone health as density.

Because it increases brittleness, fluoride can thereby actually increase the likelihood of fractures. For the body to utilize fluoride, it must be picked up from the soil in its insoluble form and absorbed by plant life before it can be assimilated. Administration of chemical fluoride actually makes teeth softer, not harder, because calcium fluoride is not as hard a structure as is calcium carbonate, the natural molecule in teeth. Nutritionist Royal Lee, D.D.S., pointed out that fluoride also inhibits and destroys vital enzymes essential for digestion and other metabolic functions. "In dilutions of one part in fifteen million, it's still poisonous enough to cut the activity of some enzymes as much as 50%." Without enzyme activity, he added, there is no life, no plant or animal that can live, so "anything that slows down enzyme activity is slowing down all life."[34] And, fluoride molecules clutch onto calcium and and magnesium and eliminate them from the body.

John Yiamouyiannis, Ph.D., an internationally recognized authority on the biological effects of fluoride, reports that fluoride is a poison, slightly more poisonous than lead and slightly less poisonous than arsenic. He adds that "A spokesperson from Proctor and Gamble, the makers of Crest toothpaste, acknowledged that a family-sized tube of fluoride toothpaste 'theoretically, at least, contains enough fluoride to kill a small child.'" Fluoride is linked to weakened immune systems, breakdown of proteins that form the structural framework (connective tissue) for skin, ligaments, muscles, bones and teeth. Fluoridated water containing as little as 1 ppm has been shown to cause genetic damage, the same level that, in animal studies, has been shown to transform normal cells into cancer cells. Gastric cancer has been associated with fluoride intake, and airborne fluoride has been linked to lung cancer.[35]

Last, a note about soft drinks, which contain three to six teaspoons of sugar each. Soft drinks are loaded with phosphorus from phosphoric acid. Phosphorus combines readily with calcium. Therefore soft drinks can draw calcium out of storage in the bones and teeth. That is how their consumption can eventually lead to osteoporosis and decayed teeth.

Reestablishing Effective Security

Dr. Versendaal has repeatedly emphasized that the key to healthy bones is good blood quality. To achieve that end, he underscores the following healing principle: "First put out the fire. Next, clean up the debris. And last, rebuild." Therefore, as Mary Jane Mack R.N., points out, "For osteoporosis, chemical reflex may be the priority before whatever else the bones need, because chemicals deplete the blood." Poor blood quality, she adds, "may or may not show up initially because you have to take care of the chemicals first."[36]

Cleaning up chemical poisons in the body begins at their port of entry: the mouth. When health practitioners find a weak reflex in the hollow of the cheek, they often recommend Parotid (SP) for chemical poisoning. Michael Smatt, D.C., who provided exactly this C.R.A.™ care for Gloria Steinem in New York City, describes what's going on. "When functioning normally, the parotid hormones stimulate the production of saliva, which neutralizes toxins and digests bacteria and chemicals before they reach the rest of the digestive system."[37] The product Parotid provides nutritional support to return these glands to peak functioning so they can clean up the toxic chemicals.[38] See Part Two, Chapter 10 for description.

After chemicals have been sufficiently eliminated, practitioners often find the body in need of essential fatty acids, because chemicals dry up the body. If this reflex point, located in the palm of each hand, is weak, they recommend Linum B6 (SP, see Part Two, Chapter 8).

The next layer of healing might then involve making certain the stomach is producing enough enzymes to break down food. If it's not, Dr. Versendaal describes how the "body will fill up fast with toxins and the person can gain 5 pounds eating one meal!" This is because fluids back up in the body. "Most people today," he continues, "have stomachs that score at a 3 [out of 10]." If this score is low, he checks for how many Zypan (SP, see previous chapter) the person needs to support digestion, and says their body size will slowly come down.

When another reflex is weak (referred to as 'metals in the liver'), practitioners know it means the person has minerals and other substances backed up in the body that need to be eliminated. When the liver can't eliminate them, the G.I. tract and kidneys become stressed because these three systems (gut-liver-kidneys) are buddies that cover for each other; if one can't get rid of a toxin, the other tries.

When all three are overwhelmed, and the body is backed up with debris and wastes, it can lead to a condition Dr. Versendaal calls 'incontinent bladder'. "There's a generation of young people who are heavy because of sick bladders," he says. "The body is supposed to discharge what it doesn't need. But the liver is overstressed with so many chemicals assaulting the body, it knocks the bladder out of commission. Then they retain fluid." This backing up of fluid can become so severe that the legs and thighs swell, and the abdomen can swell and fall, in some cases, nearly to the person's knees!

Protocols

What the body needs to prevent bone robbers, embezzlers and leachers is "a natural stream of nutritional chemistry to fuel the estimated 6 trillion chemical and electrical biological reactions that take place every second."[39] The following products are often recommended. The best results are achieved when these products are combined with outdoor exercise in fresh air and sunlight. This "brings oxygen and electrical charge in the form of ions, gives the red blood cells what they need to deliver oxygen to the body, and allows free radicals to be removed."[40]

Mary Jane Mack, R.N., sets up each person's individualized protocols, and as their body comes back to normal, she recommends they drink positively charged juices (lemonade, cranberry, cran/raspberry, pineapple/orange, etc.). Then she tests to see if they need more protein, which is often the case if their blood quality is poor. She recommends they choose foods that are 80% positive and 20% negative because that combination "charges up the body electrically."[41] Other diet recommendations depend on the person. She tries to get the body balanced first because otherwise the person's appetite will be off balance. This is especially true of big people. When their blood quality is off they fill up with water because the body's trying to protect itself."[42]

Regarding the cleansing process, Dr. Dobbins points out that when the correct product is given, the immune system starts to reset itself, and the result may be a histamine reaction. "By 48 to 72 hours they'll have the symptoms of a cold. If you don't get the histamine reaction, it's not the right one. If they feel worse, that's the right one." Although it feels like it's getting worse, it's actually a sign of getting better. To allow for that healing response, he recommends to people, "ALWAYS work your way up, doing 1 the first day, 2 the second day, 3 the third day, etc., until you get to 6."[43]

When someone is in the prodromal (initial) phase of an infection, he recommends using Organic Minerals (SP, see Part Two, Chapter 6). It supplies potassium to provide balance to the part of the nervous system that controls involuntary functions (the autonomic system). It also provides calcium in its bicarbonate form, which, as Royal Lee pointed out, is the gatekeeper for the immune system. At the first sign of a cold or anything viral, Dr. Dobbins suggests 2 Organic Minerals and 2 A and C Carbamide. If the person is becoming acutely ill, he sometimes adds Congaplex (SP, see below) to the above to support the immune system so it can prevent a secondary infection.

For best results, most practitioners recommend chewing the products at least enough to break up the binding of the tablet.

Parotid (SP) provides nutritional support for chemical poisoning. It's the product both Maureen Schaub and Sophia Tampinelli took to heal their first layer in regaining their bone health. Dr. Dobbins reports giving Parotid to one patient who "was allergic to everything. She had such a severe reaction she was absolutely laid up. She actually had to start with 1/6 of 1 Parotid a day." He points out that, in this case, "the worse the reaction, the better the result." He emphasizes how important it is to start slowly. "If you've identified the right product to help them clean out, they'll have a reaction. That gives the patient a better understanding of what's going on, and then you can lower the dose to slow down the pace of the detoxification process."

Inositol (SP) is part of the B complex of vitamins that's especially helpful for dealing with sugar cravings. It also supports the breakdown of fats.

Collagen C (SP) draws fluids from the extremities to the bladder and kidneys. Practitioners may recommend as many as 6 to 20 per day until fluid tissue levels have normalized, and then 6 a day to maintain."[44]

Cholacol (SP) is for people with severely depressed bile, as in following a cholecystectomy. It contains collinsonia root, which is a vascular astringent, often helpful for those with varicose veins. Practitioners often give 1 per meal the first day, 2 per meal the next day, 3 per meal the following day, and then back to 1, so the body can't mount a response.

Cholacol II (SP) cleans up a toxic bowel. It helps when backed up toxins create a foul intestinal gas, or a bad body odor. It helps clean people out fairly rapidly. However, points out Dr. Dobbins, there's often a liver-kidney problem underneath it which will be important to address afterwards.

Choline (SP) acts as a physiological detergent. It is also a detoxifier that supports the liver. That's why it's often recommended for episodes of acute toxicity, such as sudden food poisoning. Choline makes the bile absorb the toxins so they can be eliminated. Dr. Versendaal recommends taking several Choline (SP) tablets every 15 minutes for 3 hours for quick relief of symptoms, then several a day for a week. "Choline will enhance the liver function when the liver is poisoned . . . it will pursue and quickly neutralize bacterial chemical poisons."[45]

Spanish Black Radish (SP) is a colon detoxifying herb, especially useful in quickly eliminating toxins such as those produced by the die-off of Candida Albicans (yeast infections). It also supports the free action of the intestinal valves, the "doors" between the "rooms" of the G.I. tract so they can easily open to allow toxins to pass, and then close, so waste materials don't back-flush and retoxify the system. (See also Chapter 10.)

Dr. Dobbins adds, "Spanish Black Radish was developed to support people with colon cancer. It is for toxic bowel conditions. It's anti-parasitic, and also good for liver congestion, diarrhea, virus, and constipation. It's high in sulfluothane, which grabs cancer cells. The person may need Cholocal II also."[46]

Albaplex (SP) contains a combination of nutrients designed for kidney and liver support, especially for albuminuria (spilling of protein in the urine), which can indicate a pathological state of the kidneys, the onset of an infectious disease, or poisons in the body (either generated inside the body or from an outside source).

Immuplex (SP) provides nutrients such as B12, vitamin C, B6 and folic acid that support the immune system for the demands placed upon it by viral infections. Sometimes up to 10 a day are recommended in acute situations. It also provides nutritional factors that may be missing in people with long-standing immune deficiencies and auto-immune conditions.[47] It can be used concurrently with Congaplex (see below). Usually 3 months is a sufficient length of time to take it, but in hard cases such as fibromyalgia, which Dr. Dobbins says is a "long-term chronic viral infection, they may need Immuplex for 6 months to a year or so."[48]

Cyruta Plus (SP) helps make the bodily environment more hostile to viruses. (See Part Two, Chapter 6.)

Allerplex (SP) provides upper respiratory nutritional support, especially when reactions to toxins result in troubled breathing. It includes nutritional factors that support the adrenal glands, liver and lungs. It's often recommended for people who are food sensitive, environmentally sensitive, who suffer from asthma and other lung problems except emphysema. It's often used in conjunction with Catalyn or another immune system support.

Emphaplex (SP) provides multiple nutritional factors for support "especially for people suffering from emphysema, or lung cancer."[49]

Garlic (SP) protects against damage from free radicals that damage body tissues. It also helps maintain normal cholesterol and triglyceride levels, and a healthy flow of blood through the circulatory system. Each tablet is equivalent to one organically grown clove of whole garlic.

Thymex (SP), up to 10 a day, is often recommended for nutritional support for people who keep getting staph infections.

Congaplex (SP) provides nutritional support for people who keep getting strep infections. In acute situations, sometimes up to 20 per day are recommended. It contains a variety of nutrients to support the immune system, including calcium, as mentioned above. Since it's water soluble, it's important to spread the dosages throughout the day so it doesn't just pass out of the body. Dr. Dobbins recommends beginning to take it at the outset of feeling sick (the first prodromal phase). He says at that point, "you've got about 6 hours to get this handled, otherwise you'll be sick 10 to 14 days. Get 6 Congaplex in that 6-hour period." He adds that if you repeatedly get strep infections and have to take Congaplex, it's because you've only dealt with the acute phase; you need to rebuild your immune system with Immuplex (SP, see below).[50]

Antronex (SP) contains a natural antihistamine. It's often recommended at up to 6 a day when people develop asthma or allergies. It helps dry up the excess mucous that provides the medium in which infections can regrow. It also helps remove excess thyroxin (thyroid hormone) from the blood, so it may be suggested for people with a toxic thyroid.

Zymex (SP) is recommended for nutritional support for toxic bowel problems such as lower bowel gas, diarrhea, constipation, and for intestinal overgrowth of yeast. Zymex contributes to making an acid environment in which yeast cannot survive. It also contains enzymes that break down the yeast.[51] It frequently is combined with 3 Spanish Black Radish, 5 Cal-Amo, and 5 Lact-Enz, which contains healthy bacteria and enzymes that act as scavengers to clean up bodily pollution.

Zymex II (SP, not to be confused with Zymex), 6 per day on an empty stomach, is recommended for 8–12 weeks when parasites are a problem. It can also be used to prevent parasites when travelling to foreign countries. Because it contains factors that help digest protein, when taken on an empty stomach it digests the protein coating around the parasites.

For-Til B12 (SP), up to 6 a day, is often used in combination with 3 Cal-Amo and 3 Linum B6 for nutritional support to deal with environmental toxins (see Chapter 6).

Echinacea-C is a source of herbs and other immune system boosters, including echinacea root powder, acerola powder, rose hip powder, and vacuum dried buckwheat juice and seed. These are rich sources of calcium, copper, iron, manganese, phosphorus, potassium, B complex and bioflavonoids that also help maintain connective tissue health.

Note: After an infection, infestation or toxicity is cleared up, the body may have become deficient in lubricating oils (see Chapter 8 for protocols).

Vegetarian Protocols

STAPH OR STREP:
Echinacia-C
6 Spanish Black Radish,
3 FenGre,
3 Cal-Amo, and
3 Lact-Enz

YEAST: 6 Zymex,
3 Spanish Black Radish,
5 Cal-Amo, and
5 Lact-Enz

VIRUSES: Lomatium/Hypericum,
6 FenGre,
3 Lact-Enz,
3 Cal-Amo, and
3 Cal-Sol

PARASITES: 6 Zymex II a day on an empty stomach
for 8–12 weeks

PAROTID: 3 Cal-Sol,
3 Choline,
3 Spanish Black Radish, and
3–6 Zymex

ENVIRONMENTAL RADIATION OR ALLERGIES:
3 Linum B6,
3 Cal-Amo, and
6 Spanish Black Radish

The first five points of the Six-Point Plan for Perfect Bones covered how the bone bank develops and operates. Strengthening the security systems has provided the final component.

Now, what remains is to put these points into the actions that produce success, the focus of Part Three.

ENDNOTES

1. Mack, Author's Interview, Ibid.
2. George Higashida, President, Sun Wellness. letter to health-conscious friends, undated.
3. Shaner, Hollie, M.S.A., R.N. Interview, *NurseWeek*, April 19, 1999, p. 8.
4. Biondo, Brenda. "Are common chemicals scrambling your hormones?" in *U.S.A. Weekend*, Feb. 13–15, 1998, p. 18.
5. Gaby, Ibid., p. 16.
6. Mack, Author's Interview, Ibid.
7. Mack, Author's Interview, Ibid.
8. Versendaal, Dick, D.C., Ph.D., Seminar materials.
9. Bob LeRoy, R.D. "Major Study Results Challenge Claims for Dairy" in *Vegetarian Voice*, Autumn 1997, pp. 18–19.
10. *NIH Consensus Statement*, National Institutes of Health, Office of the Director, Volume 12, Number 4, June 6–8, 1994, p. 15.
11. Versendaal and Versendaal-Hoezee, Ibid., p. 39.
12. D. A. Versendaal, D.C., Author's Interview, Ibid.
13. Gaby, Ibid., p. 11.
14. Royal Lee, D.D.S., Ibid.
15. Jean Carper, "Eat Smart," *U.S.A. Weekend*, Nov. 6–8, 1998, p. 15.
16. West, Ibid., Vol. 15, Issue 7, July 1998, p. 6.
17. Mack, Author's Interview, Ibid.
18. Dobbins, Ibid.
19. Versendaal, Seminar materials, Ibid.
20. John Lee, M.D., *Natural Progesterone, The Multiple Roles of a Remarkable Hormone*, Ibid., pp. 81–82.
21. Dobbins, Ibid.
22. West, Ibid., Vol. 15, No. 4, p. 5.
23. NIH Consensus Statement, Ibid., p. 15.
24. Brown, Ibid., pp. 165–166.

25. Gaby, Ibid., p. 206.
26. Gaby, Ibid., p. 208.
27. Gaby, Ibid., p. 211.
28. Megan Flaherty. "Healthy Planet, Hospitals learn to clean up their act" in *NurseWeek*, Vol. 12, No. 2, Jan. 25, 1999, p. 1.
29. Warren, Author's Interview, Ibid.
30. Reported in Price Pottenger Foundation Newsletter from Acupuncture and Electro-Therapeutics Res. Int. J, 20: 133–148, 1995.
31. Dobbins, Ibid.
32. Versendaal, Seminar, Ibid.
33. Dobbins, Ibid.
34. Royal Lee, D.D.S. Ibid.
35. John Yiamouyiannis, Ph.D. "Lifesavers Guide to Fluoridation, Risks/Benefits Evaluated", a report published by the Safe Water Foundation, Delaware, Ohio, 1988, pp. 1–6.
36. Mack, Author's Interview, Ibid.
37. Michael Smatt, D.C. "Gloria Steinem" in *Today's Chiropractic*, March/April 1996, pp.76–80.
38. Versendaal, Seminar, Ibid.
39. Versendaal, Ibid.
40. Versendaal, Author's Interview, Ibid.
41. Mack, Author's Interview, Ibid.
42. Mack, Ibid.
43. Dobbins, Ibid.
44. D. A. Versendaal and Dawn Versendaal Hoeze, C.R.A.™ *and Designed Clinical Nutrition*, Ibid., p. 140.
45. Versendaal, Seminar, Ibid.
46. Dobbins, Ibid.
47. Standard Process Training Session, Ibid., p. 34.
48. Dobbins, Ibid.
49. Dobbins, Ibid.
50. Dobbins, Ibid.
51. Versendaal and Versendaal-Hoezee, Ibid., p. 26.

Part Three

CHAPTER TWELVE

Proceeding

Likely it's too late for you to build your peak bone mass, because you're probably over 20 years old. However, it's not too late for you to do something effective about assessing your bone bank status and making additional deposits if necessary. Nor is it too late to bring your account into proper balance so that what you withdraw doesn't exceed what you're depositing.

You can secure your future physical health in the same way you assure your future financial health: through the process of investing. That's why finding out you may be developing osteoporosis can turn out, like it did for me, to be a blessing in disguise. In taking the steps to turn it around, you learn how to rebuild various body systems and keep yourself in as good health as possible considering the various vicissitudes of life. You not only improve present health, but also invest in future well-being.

Dan Newell, N.C., points out that "Menopause is a great time to reevaluate what the last 50 years of your life have been. It's a great time to not just address symptoms but bring the body back into balance."[1]

Jennie deMaria is preparing to do just that. Now at age 47, she is entering her midlife phase. She has always eaten a good diet based on whole foods, and up until now, she's been in excellent health. She's had two healthy children and stayed active as an avid hiker and gardener. In the last 10 years, though, she's become more sedentary, in part because of working in an office to supplement family income. Now she fears the onset of some recent symptoms are the beginning of osteoporosis, and she doesn't want that to happen:

"After reading *Perfect Bones*, I recognized some of the characteristics of withdrawals from my bone bank, beginning some 13 years ago with broken teeth and a dark spot on my cheek. I do have the genetic predisposition: Northern European, fair skinned. I'm part Italian and part German."

Some symptoms she assumes are related to the onset of menopause: "a feeling of anxiety and feeling volatile, like anything could happen and it wouldn't be anything good. I feel not only physically fragile, but emotionally as well. I do have very brittle nails, toenails more than fingernails, for some odd reason." She's had a couple of nightsweats and her periods have changed from normal and regular to long (7 days instead of 4) and frequent (two a month). They are accompanied by headaches that started about six months ago: "I get a premenstrual headache that no aspirin or ibuprophen can take away. It starts up to five days before the onset of my period and lasts the duration of my period. It doesn't happen any other time."

Along with her hair now rapidly turning gray, she's noticed that "my lower back is always snapping in the morning. It's stiff and uncomfortable, it makes noise. When I stand up straighter I hear it snap. It lessens as the day wears on, but then I might get it again in the evening. I have a condition called `otosclerosis' (progressive deafness due to the formation of spongy bone around the stapes bone in the ear). The stapes bone in the ear has grown too large to do its job of vibrating on the drum, so I have some hearing loss in one ear. I guess the nerve is damaged." (Note: since the body robs calcium from any bone to keep blood levels up, this ear condition may have resulted from calcium being borrowed from the stapes bone. If so, and if the nerve is not permanently damaged, it's possible she could regain this hearing loss as she balances her bone bank account.)

She's also noted increasing heart palpitations. "I have a specific situation in my heart: mitral valve prolapse. I originally was diagnosed with a murmur when I was getting a physical to go to college. Later when I went for checkups when I was pregnant a doctor diagnosed it as mitral valve prolapse, so I have to take massive antibiotics when I have dental work done, but that's a problem for me because I automatically get a yeast infection. By now I've probably had ten yeast infections in the last five years." (Note: This condition is one sometimes associated with magnesium deficiency.)

Last, she adds, "I also feel like my strength in my bones in my arms and my stamina has diminished. I'm not as strong now as I was in my mid-thirties.

I know that I need to supplement my calcium intake but haven't been able to figure out what form it should be in and what minerals it should be taken in combination with so it doesn't just pass through my body and do me harm. The manuscript has given me insight and I now think there might be levels I need to take for different parts of my body to trigger natural body responses that help my bones. I now want to know what my body specifically needs. I don't trust generic, over-the-counter dosages and one-size-fits-all."

After reading *Perfect Bones*, Jenny wanted to be tested. That process revealed two of the six points that needed addressing right away: Point Four, balancing her hormonal system (specifically adrenals and pituitary), and Point Two, certain minerals, and vitamins to carry the minerals into her bones.

After these discoveries, she remarked that she was "in awe at the process of being tested. It reminds me of witnessing Aikido masters because it's similar to the remarkable things they do with the flow of energy, such as a small person overpowering a large one. I'm amazed at how sensitive the tester is to me. There's something I don't really understand that's at work here. I felt for myself how my testing arm went weak in problem areas. It's heartening to know that people can tune into the body's mysterious circuitry like this and know how to work with it.

"I feel relieved that the problems in my body have been pin-pointed. I'm eager to try the protocols and experience the effect they'll have on me."

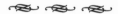

If, like Jenny, you also want to be tested, where do you locate a qualified practitioner?

ENDNOTE

1. Newell, Author's Interview, Ibid.

CHAPTER THIRTEEN

Practitioners

Health practitioners that are competent to use C.R.A.™ to assess your nutritional needs and make recommendations for your unique body are to be found in a variety of professional ranks: physicians, nurses, chiropractors, dentists, naturopaths, nutritional consultants, dieticians, and, for animals, veterinarians.

Most practitioners learned C.R.A.™ initially by experiencing the results in their own lives and then decided to undertake the training. Mary Jane Mack, R.N., for example, learned about C.R.A.™ through her horses' veterinarian. When her sick horses got better in 3 months, she decided to attend Dr. Versendaal's seminar, where she says she'd "never heard the body presented that made so much sense to me with such easy solutions. I'd worked in labor, delivery, surgical recovery, intensive care. By the end of the day I knew that's what I was going to do." She began studying, attending seminars, and gradually the word spread. She never advertised, she said. "The more I learned, the more people appeared. It was word of mouth. They came and brought their families."[1]

The health care professionals who do C.R.A.™ can be located in a variety of ways. Some practitioners are on the Internet. You can use a search engine, or enter "www.search.com" and type in "contact+reflex+analysis". A recent experience doing this yielded 96 matches.

Another way is to contact Standard Process. They are online at 'www.standardprocess.com'. You can call them at 800-558-8740 or e-mail them at 'info@standardprocess.com'. Ask who's a good, active, well trained C.R.A.™ practitioner in your area. If, when you call the recommended practitioner, they are not taking new clients, ask their office manager who that practitioner recommends.

One list of practitioners is available by sending $7 and making checks payable to:

Open Hand Trust
519 W. Mountain Ave.
Fort Collins, Co. 80521

If you follow any of these leads, you will find that many practitioners are chiropractors. Why have so many chiropractors recently turned to nutrition? Michael Dobbins, D.C., a former chiropractic college professor who now trains professionals in clinical nutrition, has an idea about that. "At the turn of the century the average diet was pretty good, so chiropractors did adjustments and people got well. But now we're not feeding cells, and correcting a nerve impulse problem won't do it."

The list of names you will compile likely will be people who are certified in Contact Reflex Analysis.™ Therefore the practitioners on your list probably (according to Jack Caputo, D.C.) use C.R.A.™ as a primary technique complementing their practice and have completed at least 40 hours of postgraduate training under the auspices of an accredited chiropractic college. Additionally, most of them continue to study C.R.A.™

Once you have some names, it's time to find the right match. Since you're going to be working with this person over time, you'll need to develop a good working relationship based on trust. Therefore, if you're the kind of person who wants a scientifically oriented practitioner, for example, you might choose someone who can recite chapter and verse of the chemical pathways of a given metabolic process. However, such rigors are unnecessary for the purpose of getting back your bones and your health. Instead, you might need to choose a practitioner who's less adept at quoting the literature, but listens and relates to you, understands your difficulties and helps you trust what they're recommending. If you need support staying on the protocols, the second type might be better for you.

Luckily, most practitioners are a mix of both. The key factor is do they know how to help you get your bones back? You will find suitable practitioners among both the scientifically oriented and the relationship oriented. Many effective clinicians have the "bedside manner" of a bull in a china shop; many who are easy to trust and relate to lack clinical skills.

To evaluate practitioners on your list, consider:

Do they have the training?

Are they C.R.A.™ certified?

Do they watch Dr. Versendaal's videos and/or attend his workshops to keep up to date?

Do they have experience?

How long have they been practicing?

How many people with osteoporosis have they helped?

Are they pushing products rather than improving your health?

Keep in mind that practitoners in one area of the country may have a different emphasis from those in another area owing to different dietary habits of the local population, regional soil and water conditions and availability of foods.

Having satisfied this level of inquiry, you'll next want to consider how the person works. Practitioners structure their appointments and fees in a variety of effective ways. On one end of the spectrum are those who have you write down your symptoms prior to the appointment, read them off when you begin your time with them, and in a few short minutes, they've adeptly and skillfully managed to test you completely and design your protocol. Their fees are also likely to be lower because they are seeing large numbers of people per hour. The advantage is that it hasn't cost you much, you have an effective protocol, and, if you do what they suggest, you're likely to see good results.

In the middle range are practitioners who take a bit more time, perhaps a half hour, and in addition to effectively assessing you, can listen to and address some of your concerns.

At the other end of the range are those who charge an hourly fee, and often integrate C.R.A.™ testing and designing your protocol into other kinds of healing work such as various forms of bodywork or counseling. This way of working allows for the greatest individual attention, and, because it requires the most time with the practitioner, may also come with the highest hourly fee.

Each way of working has its strong points. What's important is for you to know what you need to stay on the protocols and come back for reassessment at the proper time. It's no good getting a low rate on the testing fee, but then not having sufficient support to keep going. It's simply too easy to misread bodily changes as meaning something negative about the healing process. Having the point of view of your health care professional at those times is often the difference between becoming disheartened and quitting, and realizing you goal is within reach and staying the course through to victory.

Insurance coverage depends on the insurance carrier, the state in which your practitioner works, and your practitioner's professional degree and whether or not your practitioner accepts insurance payments. As of this writing, some carriers cover office visits but not the products, and a few are now considering covering products with an eye to long-term savings.

Once you've decided on a practitioner, it's time to find out which protocols are right for you.

ENDNOTE

1. Mack, Ibid.

~~ CHAPTER FOURTEEN

Protocols and Products

Once you launch your own quest for perfect bones, you're likely to be confronted by the vast array of nutritional products on the market today. Since sorting them out could take a novice an entire lifetime, a better option is to make your choices by tapping into the professional knowledge and experience of your health practitioner as well as using your own knowledge and intuition.

One of the first things you'll find is that most practitioners recommend real herbs and whole food concentrates because these products are the most likely to truly produce healing. If you're like I was, you may have to find out the hard way. Initially I'd thought the difference between synthetic chemical isolates and whole food concentrates was marginal and didn't matter. I'd recovered my bones taking whole food concentrates because that's what my practitioner recommended, and that's what Dr. Versendaal recommended. Yet my connective tissue remained weak.

In the grocery store one day, I thought I'd pick up some vitamin C. I had enough sophistication to know that if the label didn't specifically say "no lactose", that the product likely used lactose as a filler and tableting agent. (I am lactose intolerant.) I found a lactose-free product and purchased a generous-sized bottle. I took it as directed for months, during which time my alignment kept not holding (a signal of weak adrenals or weak connective tissue). I could not figure it out. Finally my local health practitioner found the culprit: the "vitamin C" product actually contained only ascorbic acid, which is one small fraction of the whole vitamin C complex. This chemical isolate can actually be harmful in higher doses. I hadn't known the difference then, but my body certainly did. I began the whole food concentrate immediately and began to heal.

A second experience—this time with synthetic vitamin B complex—convinced me. I'd begun taking it to support my heart health, but a few weeks after starting to take it, I felt worse, weaker, like my heart was working even harder. At a professional seminar I had an acoustic electrocardiogram (the same thing as an EKG, except it uses sound to translate heart patterns onto graph paper). When my synthetic vitamin B product was added to my body, the heart graph flattened! The synthetic product was depressing all my heart functions!

Synthesized chemicals that imitate one fraction of a whole food simply do not carry the healing power of a true whole food concentrated to clinical potency. That's why so many health practitioners use Standard Process products, and many use them exclusively. That's also why some scientific research projects that have studied using nutrition for healing carry such mixed results. Many of the experiments were conducted using synthetic chemical isolates instead of whole food concentrates.

One quick way to know whether the product you're considering is whole or synthetic is to read the label. You will likely recognize the names of foods and herbs, such as "beets" or "tillandsia", and will find it difficult to pronounce or comprehend words that include alpha, beta, gamma, hydroxy-, tri- etc. Also, if the product carries a patent number, it's been chemically altered, which is what makes it eligible to be patented. Whole foods cannot be patented. Again, your practitioner's expertise will guide you.

Osteoporosis, as we have seen, is a symptom, not a cause. Since each person's body is different, each plan for achieving perfect bones is specific to each individual. The wisdom of each body presents to the trained practitioner which problems to address and in what order. Trusting this innate bodily wisdom as a guide in combination with the wisdom of a health professional is central to having healthy bones.

It is this innate bodily wisdom that the C.R.A.™ practitioner is questioning during testing. Yet, if you were to be tested by several practitioners, you might find yourself confused because one recommends product A, another product B, while a third suggests a combination of C and D. This variety is an indication not of incompetence, but of the uniqueness of each practitioner's approach.

In the world of clinical nutrition, all roads can ultimately lead to Rome, meaning that the goal of perfect bone health can be approached from a variety of directions. Also, each practitioner may address the same general weaknesses with a particular emphasis, given their knowledge of products, your state of health and your priorities.

There are a number of formulations available to provide nutritional support for the hormonal system, for example, each with a slightly different makeup. One product might have an additional component to support the pancreas, for instance, while another adds nutrition for the liver. As Dr. Dobbins puts it, "To choose a product, there's so much good stuff in everything. That's why we appear to have conflicting protocols . . . but when you give good nutrition, it feeds the system and they get well."[1]

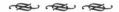

If you were to ask practitioners for some cookbook recipe for healthy bones, they'd likely all reply that what each person needs is highly individual. However, some practitioners have named particular combinations people are likely to need while still recommending that each individual be personally evaluated.

Dr. Royal Lee, D.D.S., recommended a general protocol that included ionizable calcium, raw bone enzyme protein factors, sex hormone precursors, prothrombin factor, potassium and trace mineral source, and calcium diffuser. Per day, he suggested:[2]

3 Cyro-Yeast
6–12 Calcium Lactate
2 tsp. Calcifood or 3 Biost
3 Chlorophyll Complex
1 Organic Minerals
1 Cataplex F

Dr. Versendaal, for example, has said that if someone were to take only one product for improving their bone health, that one "would be e-Poise (SP) because it builds blood, and blood builds bone." E-poise was originally designed from recommendations by George Goodheart, D.C., who founded the healing system of Applied Kinesiology™. E-Poise contains a multitude of nutrients the body needs: iron, vitamins, enzymes, herbs, essential fatty acids, etc. The combination of nutrients in e-Poise makes contributions to many of the points of the six point plan for good bone health, including good blood quality and overall endocrine balance and support. If given enough time, Dr. Versendaal states, e-Poise can provide what bones need. That's why e-Poise is likely to be recommended for young people looking for a good preventive product while they are still in relatively good health. As Dr. Michael Dobbins emphasizes, "There's benefit in a small amount long-term for maintenance also."[3]

Mary Jane Mack, R.N., notices that "Most people on whom I pick up osteoporosis have been depleted in their blood for a long time, so they need e-Poise. That's the important preventive because it builds the blood and supports the bones. Without vitamins and iron the bones become weak and can swell. That's what causes pain and makes a lot of people worry about their bones. Pain is their presenting complaint. Some people complain of achy joints, adjustments that don't hold . . . underneath they're deficient in vitamins and iron."[4]

However, many people are too far out of balance or too short on time to use e-Poise alone. Then, to hit the problem (of poor blood quality and poor bone health) from all angles, Dr. Versendaal recommends, per day for adults (all Standard Process products):

1 Calcifood Wafer
1 E-Poise
1 Chlorophyll Complex Perle
1 Cataplex F Perle
1 Utrophin (female) or 1 Prost-X (male)
1 Mammary (female)
1 Ovex (female) or 1 Orchic (male)
1 Zypan, to aid digestion and absorption

When the person is even further out of balance, in severe cases he has recommended 3 times the above dosages a day for 3 months or until well recovered, then to maintain at one per day of each.

Mary Jane Mack, R.N., who has used this protocol with some of her clients, comments: "Using this protocol for osteoporosis, people are doing even better [than before it was devised]. People turn around faster, they notice a difference sooner. In 12 weeks you see big differences. It depends on what their state of health is. If you have to clean up deficiencies in the body first it could take 6 months to a year. For example, things will go more slowly if you need to clean up chemicals or other things like bacteria that are weakening the system."[5]

If the person has or is prone to gout, Dr. Versendaal takes a different approach, which is to take, 3 times a day:

2 Cataplex F Perles
2 Min-Tran
2 Chlorophyll Complex
2 Zypan

However, if he discovers someone needs more than 3–5 e-Poise a day, he would use a strategy with a different emphasis:

2 Lact-Enz
1 e-Poise
1 Organic Iodine
1 Min-Tran
3 A C Carbamide
2 Betafood
2 Zypan
1 Chlorophyll Complex

The emphasis of this protocol is designed to help the cells eliminate toxins and take in nutrition.[6]

Bruce West, D.C., whose newsletter *Health Alert* reaches thousands of subscribers, brings together a protocol with the following combinations:

Biost, 6 a day
CalMa Plus, 3 a day
Calcifood Wafers or Biodent, 6–12 a day.

If the person has involvement in the mandible (jaw bone), teeth or other bones of the face, he'd likely use Biodent in place of Calcifood Wafers.

For vegetarians, Dr. West would likely include:

Calcium lactate, 6 per day, and
Chlorophyll Complex, 2–3 per day.

He emphasizes, "Each patient is different. The above are cookbook recipes only. He adds that he uses Standard Process products in part because "The way they design their products, they stimulate and normalize hormones."[7]

Dr. Michael Dobbins says that if he were to use only one product, he would choose Ferrofood (SP). "Ferrofood is the finest blood-building product on the market. Ferrous lactate doesn't constipate, it's far more assimilable. The body doesn't eliminate what it needs. Ferrofood contains bone meal, and nutritional support for the duodenum, spleen, adrenals, stomach, and liver."[8]

And, for dealing with bone pain, nutritionist Royal Lee, D.D.S., states it is often due to lack of raw food vitamins and amino acids, particularly lysine and tryptophane, that are affected by heat such as pasteurization, cooking and autoclaving.[9] He recommends:

3 Catalyn or 6 CyroFood
3–6 Biost
1 Protefood
6 Prostex

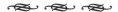

Your practitioner will help you decide what your body needs. During your appointment, communicate clearly about your priorities. Is your current goal, for example, to chase down a symptom that's been bothering you, or are you interested in general health improvement, or are you looking for a personalized program for improving your bone health? Your practitioner can design a protocol according to the priorities your body reveals or create one designed to address a particular symptom, and the two may not be the same. Many practitioners will ask you to bring in a pre-written list of what you want, the better to serve your goals.

Once you have your practitioner's recommendations, it's time to make some decisions about what products to purchase. You might decide to purchase those that address a particular symptom that's been bothering you, or to purchase the ones, if different, that address the top priorities your body revealed during the testing.

For most people, economic considerations play a role in making such decisions. To determine what a protocol might cost, you can ask your practitioner for a price list so you can refer to it as needed. Remember that, even if your body revealed 5 or 6 or even

10 weaknesses in need of nutrition, nonetheless that's far too much for the body to correct at one time. Even if you're enthusiastic and want everything corrected right now, your practitioner will no doubt recommend that you address no more than the top 3 priorities. There's no point in overdoing it as the body can't deal with too much at a time.

Having narrowed down your choices, next consider how many pills that will mean you need to take each day. Your final decision about what to take will be affected both by how many pills you can realistically take each day, and how much they will cost. If you have a hard time taking pills, and if economic considerations are primary, you are better off to start by addressing the top priority only. Getting that protocol into your body will give you the nutrition that's most important now, and will also start to take some stress off other organs and systems that have been attempting to fill in. You will obtain the best results by taking the products to correct one weakness for three full months rather than taking products to correct three weaknesses and taking them only for a month.

Having made your choices about products and protocols, you are ready to begin the healing process.

ENDNOTES

1. Dobbins, Ibid.
2. Lee, Royal, D.D.S. *Therapeutic Food Manual*, Ibid., p. 219.
3. Ibid.
4. Mack, Ibid.
5. Ibid.
6. Versendaal, Seminar materials, Ibid.
7. West, Author's Interview, Ibid.
8. Dobbins, Ibid.
9. Lee, Ibid.

⇜ CHAPTER FIFTEEN

The Process of Healing

Fresh from your practitioner, strengthened with new information and armed with your own personal protocol, you are ready for a most important step: using your emotional backbone in your quest for perfect bones. In other words, it's time to exercise the part of yourself that can stand independently, that can be firm and resolute. You'll need a solid commitment that you will do whatever it takes to keep or regain your bone health. In this instance, a strong emotional backbone in the form of personal resolve precedes a sound physical one.

Few people lose their bone health over a short period of time, and few regain it that way. Taking nutritional protocols is not like taking a pain pill or an antibiotic where you feel the difference immediately. What you are undertaking is the remodelling and upgrading of the basic structures that make up your bodily cells—especially those of your bones. It would be most unusual for you to notice big changes within a short time-span. More than likely, the process of regaining bone health, or even preventing poor bone health, will take several visits to a competent practitioner. And in between those visits, it will mean your staying on the protocols for three months, making it a new habit to take these products daily.

Some people run into difficulty because they don't like to swallow pills. A couple things help here. One is to remember that you are swallowing food, not medicine. Think of your protocols like part of your meal, and include them with your breakfast, lunch and dinner. Second, if you don't like to take pills, you can open the capsules and sprinkle the contents into your juice or cereal or other food. If the protocol includes tablets, you can crush them into a fine powder with the side of a butter knife. Then add the powder to your juice or food.

If you're not at home for some meals, you can keep a small stock of your protocol in your desk at work, your briefcase or purse. You can put the pills for one meal in a small container such as a plastic bag so they're all ready. In the beginning, it will take a little extra effort to get things set up, but once you make the habit, it will be no trouble at all. Keep your long-term goal in mind. See yourself as having perfect bones and being able to remain healthy and active.

No series of nutritional protocols can promise to extend your life by even so much as one nanosecond. What good nutrition can do is help prevent the foreshortening of that lifespan. Good nutrition can also support your having the best possible health while you're here.

In deciding whether to follow such a program for yourself, you have to weigh what that quality of life is worth to you and what you and your loved ones might stand to lose if you don't undertake this healing work. Weigh the personal cost of your being unable to work and of requiring others' services to care for you against the money it will cost you to do the protocols and the quality of life you stand to keep and even gain. That puts things in a perspective that makes clear the implications of the choice you make.

Too, we all want to be taken care of sometimes. That's why it helps to consider how much your temptation not to take your protocols is influenced by a desire to be taken care of. Once you're clear about that, you can come up with ways you could arrange to be taken care of without having to lose your bones and your health.

As someone whose bone health has been so poor that I had no other choice but to be taken care of by others, I can tell you from personal experience, even when kind, loving, and supportive people are your caregivers, it's no picnic. I'd much rather be pain-free and able to function. Nobody else can take care of you the way you can!

You may indeed feel overwhelmed at first, but it's really not that hard. Yes, you'll have to stick to it on a daily basis, but you have to stick to breathing and eating on a daily basis, and you've managed. Once you figure out what the new habits are and start doing them, they'll become just as automatic as eating and breathing, and you'll find yourself growing stronger every day. This increased physical strength will in turn motivate your emotional resolve and keep you going.

Just take the step that's right in front of you to do, and once that's done, take the next one that's right in front of you. That's the way you'll reach your goal with a minimum of fuss and a maximum of results. Assume there will be times you feel like quitting, and arrange in advance to talk with supportive people . . . your family, your practitioner or friends. Then when you feel downhearted, let them know, and ask them to remind you that healing your bones is an organic process; that you didn't get this way overnight and you won't regain perfect health overnight either.

You lose your health, not in one giant leap, but slowly, in phases over the years. That is likely to be the same way you will regain your health. It's unusual to get back to perfect health, especially healthy bones, in one fell swoop. You'll need to stick with it. If you forget a dose or go off your protocol for awhile, don't use that as an excuse. It's not too late. Don't lose another day, just get back on it.

However, if something feels "not right" about your protocol, let your practitioner know so that adjustments can be made. Trust that your intuition is telling you something important, and get the help you need to find out what it is and get back on track.

Still, you may wonder how long this whole healing process will take. The nature of the skeleton is that it is designed to repair itself with fresh atoms every three months. The process you are going to undertake, then, is to bring your actions into alignment with this process. That's the big picture. You don't have to know anything fancy or get a degree in biochemistry, or become a research scientist. People kept their bones healthy long before science was invented. You are simply going to aid your body to do what it already does naturally. And, because this repair process is undertaken and completed on a three-month timetable, you can use each season to heal the next layers indicated by your body. And, as you do so, you'll be bringing your whole body, not just your bones, closer and closer to optimum health.

How long will this repair process likely be? Bruce West, D.C., answers: "For the typical 65-to 75-year old women who've been osteoporotic, its likely to be 6 months before strength returns and 18 to 24 months before they're approaching normalcy."[1] He adds that when osteoporosis suffers have all the factors in place, including taking the right protocols for them, eating a proper diet including lots of raw foods, and exercising, that they then "can look forward to relief and feeling 20 years younger within 8 to 18 months."[2]

However long it takes for you, you will obtain the best results by working closely with a qualified practitioner, taking the clinical nutrition protocols that are right for you and taking them in the order that's right for you. You may not need to address all six points. Your practitioner will help you find out all that.

Last, remember the process of clinical nutrition is one of slow and steady physical rebuilding, and requires patiently working in concert with nature's timetable. Nature knows how to make perfect bones; your job is to provide what is needed to support that process.

Where Are They Now?

This book would not be complete without coming back to the people whose stories fill its pages. Such revisiting puts a human face on the healing process and highlights its natural ups and downs—information that can provide much needed support for staying the course.

Since the dramatic demonstration that my own bone health had come crashing down in the airport lounge, I have needed to take protocols that address all six layers of the plan for perfect bones. This has even entailed taking some more than once, as when I switched brands of vitamin C, acquired weak collagen fibers and had to rebuild my connective tissue again. Although not what I'd have chosen, this experience was one that taught me the importance of taking whole food concentrates rather than synthetic isolates.

When I began to rebuild, I was exhausted and frail. Overexertion was defined by narrow parameters such as leaning over to brush my teeth in the morning, or walking to the corner and back. Now it's defined by hiking and swimming for hours at a time too many days in a row!

I intend to continue being tested periodically and taking whatever whole food concentrates are indicated. I know from personal experience that not just my bones, but my whole body benefits. I have come to believe that this is the best health insurance there is.

We first met Carol Gieg in Chapter 1, where she revealed that she had suffered numerous bone fractures before the age of 22. In Chapter 3, she recounted her journey through the treatment options offered her by some 10 different physicians. She has addressed weaknesses relating to Point One, connective tissue; Point Two, minerals and vitamins; Point Three, essential fatty acids and the gallbladder support for metabolizing them. She is now addressing, Point Four, hormones for bones.

Her situation is an example of someone who has required longer times on the protocols to strengthen her systems. Her poor bone health is one of the most long-standing kinds. It is a likely guess, given the information available from her medical history and C.R.A.™ testing, that she experienced follicular shutdown at an early age—a condition in which the corpus luteum of the ovum is unable to produce sufficient progesterone. It is a notoriously difficult condition to reverse.

Nonetheless, C.R.A.™ testing shows considerable improvements in all her scores. She continues a vitally active lifestyle which includes hiking, biking and canoeing regularly. She has suffered no additional fractures. She reports feeling that her body has some reserves now, that her hair has started growing again, and that she feels like her body could take over natural hormone production now. "Even if I don't improve from here," she emphasizes, "the improvement in my health is significant."

A bone mineral density test taken soon after her improved C.R.A.™ test scores showed some improvement. However, she knows that BMD studies only reveal bone density, which is one part of the equation for healthy bones. The other part—suppleness rather than brittleness—will not be revealed in these tests.

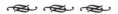

We met Edith Crenshaw in Part One, Chapter 3, where she was contending with the various medical options to deal with her unhealthy hip and shoulder bones. Currently Edith has been so busy taking care of her dying husband that she hasn't even been able to consider the hip replacement surgery her doctor recommended. Now, having seen what her husband has gone through with his failing bone health, it is doubtful that she ever will want to have the surgery. Perhaps when she completes the process of taking over management of her husband's financial and legal affairs, she may decide to pursue a nutritional approach. Her daughter is encouraging her in that direction.

We were introduced to layers of healing by Sophia Tampinelli. Not long after being tested, she had what she refers to as "a

$6,000 screw" placed in her 5th metacarpal (knuckle of the hand) because she'd fractured it after falling on the street. She'd also suffered a compression fracture of T4 (thoracic spine bone). After that, she says that she began to realize her health was so poor because of the stresses of her life. She has since made some major changes, including her employment situation. She's now had enough experience taking her C.R.A.™ protocols that she's begun to learn what she needs to do to make her health better.

She's encountered a common difficulty, however. She reports, "What I found out is that I need to be consistent about my protocol because when I start to feel better, I forget to take it, and then I slide right back. It's like antibiotics, when you feel better you don't finish the whole bottle. And when I feel bad, I feel too tired to take them. I have to will myself into taking them. At this point, I'm much more committed to doing it."

Renee Freeman, who takes care of Berle Johns, you may recall, had told Berle that if she didn't take her C.R.A.™ protocol, she, Renee, would refuse to take care of her. Berle took the pills, which addressed Point Two, minerals and their vitamin helpers. Renee reports that following her compressed back fracture, Berle, now 83, took massive doses for 4 months and then went on maintenance. The following January Berle was checked by a doctor and everything was OK.

In March of 1998, though, Berle fell and fell hard, right on her hip bone. The paramedics came and took her to the hospital. They were certain she'd broken her hip. Since the local hospital found nothing on x-ray, they sent her to a big city hospital, thinking their own equipment wasn't sophisticated enough. But there was no fracture, only bruising. Says Renee, "I just know she didn't have a fracture because of the maintenance doses she's been taking. Luckily, she's faithful about taking those pills."

The little miniature dachshund, Lulu, who taught me so much about the role of essential fatty acids in physical and emotional health, is no longer with us. After a long and active life, she finally died of old age. She had remained able to take long hikes, keeping up with the pace of brisk-walking, two-legged companions until shortly before she died.

Once she had come out of her EFA deficit, with its concomitant depression, she regained both her dynamic personality and her physical flexibility. Her recovery is one of the best examples of the power of clinical nutrition to heal, for she had no other agenda except to behave the way she felt. When she was in pain and felt awful, she showed it directly. And when the pain was gone and she was in robust health, she demonstrated it—expressing her wants, desires, opinions and zest for life in a variety of endearing ways.

Crystal M. shared her story about the role of gallbladder health and essential fatty acids in Part Two, Chapter 8. To promote her healing process, she has combined a C.R.A.™ approach, input from health practitioners using other nutritional approaches, products purchased over-the-counter, and some prescriptions recommended by physicians.

Her initial C.R.A.™ visit revealed a host of nutritional deficits covering all Six Points. She's had the least health difficulty with Point One, connective tissue. For Point Two, Minerals, she has taken protocols to correct mineral imbalances, especially ones that made her body alkaline. But the first weakness she addressed was Point Three, Essential Fatty Acids. As you may recall, she took protocols to support her body in dissolving gallstones, and to aid her bile production. Then she was able to begin metabolizing essential fatty acids, which her body desperately needed.

After raising her EFA levels, she began to address Point Four, hormone imbalances involving her adrenals, parathyroids, hypothalamus, thyroid gland and sex hormone levels. As her hormonal system began to reactivate, she experienced a period of hot flashes.

Her healing process has also included metabolic support for digesting proteins (Point Five), as well as addressing numerous environmental allergies, toxins in her liver, and parasites (Point Six).

According to bone density studies, her bone health was severely compromised when she began this process. Like Carol Gieg, it is likely Crystal also experienced follicular shutdown at a young age. At one point she had weighed under 70 pounds as a result of environmental allergies. Although she is still in the process of balancing her hormonal system, her C.R.A.™ scores have improved significantly. She has continued to resist pressure by her physician to take Fosamex. As of this writing, she is about to have another bone mineral density study.

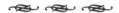

John G., you may recall, had low sex hormone levels as a result of surgical treatment for prostate cancer, which, his doctor said, had disappeared completely after 2¼ months on C.R.A.™ protocols for yeast and virus. Despite this victory, John did not continue being tested, nor did he stay on any other protocols. A couple of years after his recovery from cancer, he developed Parkinson's to the point where it was difficult for him to move from one room to the next, let alone get himself to a C.R.A.™ appointment in a neighboring town.

Nonetheless, he was C.R.A.™ tested at age 81, a few years after his surgery, which revealed that he was low in essential fatty acids, that his immune system was not working properly, that he was very low in sex hormones, and that his bone health was very poor. He did not take any further protocols.

A few months later, John's doctor told him his cancer had recurred. A few months after that, he fell and broke his hip. During the surgery to repair it, his surgeon remarked that John's hip bone was like powder. His surgeon ground up the powdery bone and put it back in with wires because he thought John wouldn't survive hip replacement surgery. Afterwards John fell again, which necessitated the hip replacement surgery. Then he fell a third time, causing his hip joint to come out of the socket entirely and stick out under the skin. One of his caregivers remarked that in 17 years of taking care of people, he had never seen such unmanageable pain. John did not recover from the surgery, and died six weeks after his original fall.

John's surgeon's comment about the state of John's bone health certainly verified the C.R.A.™ test findings. John's story puts one personal face on the growing numbers of old people who fracture their hips and die. One can only wonder what might have happened had he been able to take the C.R.A.™ protocols his body revealed he needed. Would he have lived longer? Probably not. Would he have continued functioning longer and suffered less? We'll never know.

Nonetheless, his story points to the need for programs and services that would make the power of clinical nutrition easily available to this population. If sufficient research findings were available to doctors, if insurance covered clinical nutrition, and if senior citizen care programs provided support for taking clinical nutritional products as well as medications, this story may have had a different outcome. No doubt we all stand to benefit by making C.R.A.™ and clinical nutrition available to this population, whom we are all slowly joining.

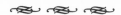

Maureen Schaub is the beautician whose involvement with C.R.A.™ began with addressing the chemical poisons she is exposed to at work. C.R.A.™ protocols, she says, put her soundly back in the game of life. The magic combination for her bones was 6/4/3: Point Six, A clean environment (toxins from work and virus); Point Four, Hormones, especially thyroid, adrenals, pituitary); and Point Three, essential fatty acids.

Checking with her a year after her first interview, she said she continues to take Parotid (SP) because she continues to be exposed to chemicals at work. "I stayed with it because I kept getting headaches before and that helped keep my lungs clear of chemicals which were contributing to the headaches . . . it helps keep the heavy feeling in my chest away that I used to get."

She also continues to take Cal-Ma Plus, along with Linum B6 to help it absorb into her bones. "When I stand on my feet all day at work, I don't go home at the end of the day feeling so fatigued."

She says that deciding to follow through with the protocols was a learning process. "I went through a lot of feelings at first, thinking it was voodoo, or a crock, because of what you're always taught. That's why my husband is skeptical. He began a protocol, started to feel better, and quit halfway through. About a year later all his symptoms came back. Some people are skeptical and have to learn."

She explains, "I took the protocols for 3 months and felt a lot better, then went off them and slowly started to feel worse again. Plus, I was worried about not getting enough calcium because I can't have dairy. It is tempting to go off the protocol when you feel good, you think you don't need it, but then you start feeling bad again and realize you need to get back on it."

She adds, "I've had better success going to C.R.A.™ practitioners than doctors, so I want to stay with it. With C.R.A.™ they want to work with you and get to the core of the problem, whereas with the doctor they're medicating you but not really getting to the core of it. I took my daughter before puberty when she had some illnesses, and they got to the core of it. She went through puberty with no problems, even though she'd had hives, allergic reactions to chemicals, smells, artificial colors, preservatives. The doctors kept suppressing it with antihistamines. If she ends up getting sick now, it's something emotional. She's 15 now, and when she gets growing pains we give her Calcium Lactate (SP) or Cal-Ma Plus and Linum B6, whatever I have in the house, and it takes the crampiness away. Her bones test strong now, and they weren't when she was first tested. Her body was so fatigued from everything the doctors were giving her."

She adds, "My own bones are the same way, they test strong too. They were in terrible shape before, and that concerned me a lot because my grandmother had osteoporosis."

Even though she doesn't have much extra money, Maureen continues to go regularly to be checked for any necessary changes, and she takes her children. She says that for her, "feeling better is priceless. I would rather spend the money and know I feel good and am taking care of myself and my future. I want a healthy life in my senior years too. I don't want to go through the pain my grandmother went through."

She says she was "really sold from the time I saw my daughter getting better. When I think about how I used to feel, I don't ever want to go back to how I used to feel. I want to move forward with my health. My health is really good now, and I want to get it even better. My goal is to get off synthetic thyroid medication entirely. My husband is still skeptical," she says, "but he's coming around I think, from seeing our experiences."

Jennie deMaria wanted to be C.R.A.™ tested after reading part of the manuscript for *Perfect Bones*. Six months later, she was retested and sent this note about it: "My initial awestruck impression of Contact Reflex Analysis™ did again surface because the analysis was so immediate and exactly pertinent to my state of being. My brain was tired, my sex hormones were very low, plus I ignored my lactose intolerance at lunch and the practitioner was able to pinpoint all of these things within 5 minutes even though we had not seen each other for 6 months."

The first testing revealed Jennie needed to address Point 4, Hormones for Bones, and Point 2, minerals and their helper vitamins. After that initial test, Jennie patched together her own version of the recommended protocols from various remedies she already had at home, had heard about through friends, or could put together from dietary intake.

The second testing revealed she was still weak on adrenals and sex hormones. She remarked, "I've known my sex hormones were low, I actually have a local uncomfortableness and my sex drive is low right now, so it's not a surprise at all. I've known all along that I haven't addressed my calcium, I'm impatient with myself for ignoring it. The testing reaffirmed what I know."

"One of the many things I am thankful for in this world is second chances. Even though the analysis came through the practitioner's hands, my physical health is in my own hands...I intend to share the knowledge of some of these supplements with my daughter who is nineteen and to encourage her to start using them. I may not have made deposits into a college fund for her (she is doing that herself) but I can try to make sure her calcium fund has plenty in it for her middle age...I am making a concerted effort to add these supplements to my diet...I hope to discern an improvement in my well being and have another C.R.A.™ test to prove it in three months."

Jennie's process reminds me of what I went through initially after being tested. Like Jennie, I thought I could get some of what I needed to strengthen weak systems through diet, or through synthetic products. I had to learn by trial and error, and that process taught me that whole foods are healing, and whole food concentrates are often necessary to complete the job. Jennie is doing the right thing to educate herself, make her own decisions and find out whether or not her body responds. Luckily, she has time to do this, for she is only in middle age, and her health is fairly good.

Now, It's Your Turn

Collectively these people's experiences demonstrate that those who continue to take their protocols, get retested and take the next protocol for their subsequent layer of healing are constantly improving their overall health and moving further and further along in their quest for perfect bones. For Berle, the process was quick and dramatic. For Carol and Crystal, it has been slower as they deal with long-standing deficits and many layers of healing. The idea that bone health is regainable is not merely an optimistic point of view, however. What some have done, others can do. Their experiences also demonstrate that catching deficits early means being able to turn them around in a shorter length of time.

Once deficits are addressed, the system for which they were intended may not need any more extra nutritional support. Or, perhaps it will need minimal support. That such maintenance doses may be required has everything to do with the modern world in which we live. Our food supply is grown on leached-out, pesticide-filled soil. Then it is adulterated with fake fats, artificial sweeteners, sprays, colors and waxes, and now, genetic engineering. This health-robbing state of affairs flourishes where governmental policies work for the profit margins of pharmaceutical conglomerates rather than for the public health. The idea, therefore, that osteoporosis has its roots in politics is not as far-fetched as it may seem.

Given that this is the modern predicament, it requires a modern solution. To feed yourself well, to have the vitality that should be your birthright when foods are adulterated and soils depleted, can indeed require the addition of foods concentrated to clinical potency.

Adulterated food in combination with the modern fixation that thin is better can prove lethal for well-being, especially that of bones. A great deal of skill and know-how are required to locate, prepare and consume foodstuffs of sufficient quality that contain real nutrients to keep one at top health. Our earliest for-bearers were able simply to reach up and pick such fruits off the tree, or dig succulent tubers from a rich and fragrant earth. Their threats to survival came, not from the supermarket or fast food restaurant, but from tigers or bears, or warring neighbors.

Modern people have traded these ills for the relative security of homes, jobs, money, purchasing power, and the comforts provided by mass culture. Now we must learn to deal with the threats hidden within this lifestyle, particularly the bone-leaching consequences of environmental toxins and allergens, foods that are devoid of the nutrition they used to contain, and other such stresses inherent in modern life.

To do so requires a proactive stance. No longer can we rest assured that our health is automatically taken care of by consuming modern foodstuffs, which in some cases have become like the Trojan horse. That big, beautiful, ripe red apple looks great on the outside, but oh, what it may contain! That local fast food restaurant may be convenient and appear inexpensive; however, those who make it their regular fare will also have to count the hidden inconveniences and expenses down the line: a gradual loss of vitality, failing health and the expenses of being unable to work.

If you feel hopeless because your mother or grandmother had osteoporosis, and you think you must carry the gene, think again. Even if there were a gene for osteoporosis, the expression of all genes, including such a (theoretical) gene, is profoundly influenced by nutritional status.

And if you like some foods that are less than optimal, don't worry. Certainly the occasional consumption of fast foods can be tolerated with minimum negative effects by a healthy person. The people most likely to be able to tolerate it are those who consistently consume a diet composed of a wide variety of fresh, whole, and generally organic foods, at least some of them raw. The key is to make the consumption of sub-optimal foods relatively rare, and to consume no or a very limited intake of sugar, white flour and refined foods. Introduction of these non-foods into the Western diet results in increased dental caries, alveoli (tooth sockets), bone degeneration and skeletal deformities, a fact discovered by Westin Price, D.D.S., in his landmark study of diet and disease.[3]

For myself, I've decided to continue to be tested and to take care of weaknesses while they're still small. I want to do whatever I can to assure that I'll live until I die. Besides, I know how I feel when all my testing scores are at a 10, and that's how I want to live if possible. So if taking a few supplements a day does that for me, it's a small price to pay.

And now, what will you decide? Whatever your choice, your bones will benefit to the extent that you apply what you've learned in these pages. No doubt your process of healing will be different from those reported here. The essential message of this book has been that there is a process of healing, that it is known, and that there is such a process for you, too.

The point is to provide a better solution to the body's need to maintain homeostatic balance than osteoporosis. This book has covered the six essential factors that can provide that better solution.

As you undergo your own bone-healing journey, you will also be making your contribution to a healthier society for us all. The information presented in this book is dedicated to that purpose.

ENDNOTES

1. West, Author's Interview, Ibid.
2. West, Ibid., Vol. 15, No. 9, p. 6.
3. Price, Westin. *Nutrition and Physical Degeneration*, Price Pottenger Nutritional Foundation, La Mesa, Ca., 1939.

✍ Glossary

acid: Any substance containing hydrogen replaceable by metals, yielding hydrogen ions as the only positively charged ions when dissolved in water

acid-base balance: In metabolism, the balance of acid to base (alkaline ash) necessary to keep the blood neutral (slightly alkaline), between pH 7.35 and pH 7.43. Minerals found in food and stored in bone play a crucial role in keeping this balance

acid ash diet: Diet that produces an acid ash when metabolized, often accomplished by decreasing fruits, vegetables and milk

alkaline: Having the reactions of a metallic hydroxide that has the property of combining with an acid to form a salt, or with an oil to form a soap

alkaline ash diet: One consisting of a normal amount of protein with moderate salt restriction

amenorrhea: Absence of menstruation

anaphylactic shock: An acute, life-threatening form of shock resulting from an allergic reaction

anovulatory: Cessation or suspension of ovulation

anticholinergic: A class of drugs used to treat the side effects of several groups of drugs in psychiatry

arthralgia: Joint pain

asphyxia: A state of suspended animation due to interference with the oxygen supply of the blood

autonomic nervous system: The involuntary or self-controlling part of the nervous system concerned with controlling involuntary functions such as glands, smooth muscle tissue and the heart. Also called the sympathetic nervous system

calcification: Deposit of lime salts in the tissues, normally in bone

cholesterol: A crystalline substance that is soluble in fats. It is a required component to build cell membranes, sex hormones and certain digestive processes. It is naturally present in the brain, nervous tissue, blood, liver (where about $1/5$ of it is manufactured) and bile. It is the largest component of gallstones

collagen: A substance existing in various tissues of the body, as in the white fibers of connective tissue. The protein prepared from connective tissue (tendons, etc.) from which gelatin is made

connective tissue: That which connects or binds together; one of the four main tissues of the body. After embryonic connective tissue becomes adult, it is found in vascular tissues such as blood and lymph, fibrous tissues, cartilage and bone. These tissues support bodily structures, bind parts together, store food, and play a role in blood formation and some defensive mechanisms

C-section or cesarean section: Surgical removal of the fetus from the womb

co-factors: Additional nutrients and enzymes needed to completely metabolize and use a given nutrient

collagen: An elastic living matrix made up of protein

corticosteroid: Hormones produced by the adrenal glands

desiccated: Products made from a concentrate of the whole gland, such as desiccated adrenal or desiccated parathyroid

ectoderm: The outer layer of cells in a developing embryo, from which develop skin structures (including the gut), the nervous system, organs of special sense, the pineal and part of the pituitary and suprarenal glands

electrical charge: The quantity of positive, negative or neutral energy present in a tissue, expressed chemically as valence, and caused by the motion of protons, neutrons and electrons, and manifesting as attraction, repulsion or magnetic forces

endocrine: Organs or glands that secrete substances such as hormones

entoderm: The innermost layer of cells in a developing embryo from which arise the epithelium of the digestive tract and its associated glands, the respiratory organs, bladder, vagina and urethra

enzyme: An organic compound capable of breaking down a substance into its component parts

fatty acids: A variety of organic acids from which fats or oils are made. Essential ones are those whose absence in the diet leads to loss of weight, eczematous skin conditions and kidney disorders

hormone: A chemical substance originating in an organ, gland, or part, which is conveyed through the blood to another part of the body, stimulating it to increased functional activity and increased secretion

hydroxyapatite: The crystals in bone made of collagen and mineral deposits in combination

hypogonadal: Low sex hormone producing

hypertension: High blood pressure, often the result of narrowing of the blood vessels, due in part to calcium formation on the vessel walls

hysterectomy: Surgical removal of the uterus, sometimes includes oophorectomy also, which is removal of the ovaries

ligament: A band or sheet of strong, fibrous connective tissue connecting the ends of bones, serving to bind them together and to facilitate or limit motion, to support visceral organs, to connect bones, cartilage, muscles and other structures

mesoderm: The middle primary germ layer of the developing embryo from which arise all connective tissues, muscular, skeletal, circulatory, lymphatic and urogenital systems and the linings of the body cavities

micronized progesterone: (natural) An exact chemical duplicate of the progesterone that is produced by the human body. Derived from extracts of yams and soybeans

mineral: Any class of substances occurring in nature, usually comprising inorganic substances, as quartz, feldspar, etc., of definite chemical composition and usually of definite crystal structure, but sometimes also including rocks formed by these substances as well as certain natural products of organic origin, as asphalt, coal, etc. Any substance that is neither animal nor vegetable.

nutraceutical: A food product or herb that has been changed slightly in its molecular structure so that it can be classified as a drug and patented

oophorectomy: Surgical removal of the ovaries

osmosis: A process that allows for elements contained in solution to pass through cell membranes so they can be used for cell metabolism or carry out products of elimination

osteitis deformans: A chronic, slowly progressive bone disorder, in which an initial phase of decalcification and softening is followed by calcium deposition with thickening, abnormal architecture, and deformity. Also called Paget's disease

osteoblast: Bone cell that forms new bone

osteoclast: Bone cell that resorbs old bone

osteocyte: A living bone cell that can become an osteoclast or an osteoblast

osteogenesis: The formation and development of bone that takes place in connective tissue or cartilage

osteogenesis imperfecta: A Latin term referring to the imperfect formation and development of bone due to defective collagen, causing bones to fracture easily. Some experts consider it a genetic disorder; others a nutritional one relating to protein in connective tissue

osteoid: The non-cellular collagenous matrix of bone

osteoporosis: Diminished structural integrity of the skeleton, including decreased bone mass, involving loss of both mineral and protein matrix components of bone

osteomyelitis: Bone infection resulting from pyogenic micro-organisms

otosclerosis: Progressive deafness due to the formation of spongy bone around the stapes bone in the ear

perimenopausal: The time surrounding menopause when many hormone changes occur

pH: a symbol used to express the degree of acidity or alkalinity of a solution. Neutral pH is 7; stomach juices are often 1.0 to 1.3; blood plasma is 7.3 to 7.5

prodromal: The initial phase of getting sick, especially with an infection

prostaglandin: A substance resembling a hormone that regulates various body processes, especially those that reduce inflammation

phylogenetic: Concerning the development of a race or group

phytochemicals: Whole nutrients contained in plants

phytoestrogen: Plant sources of estrogen or substances from which estrogen is made

preeclampsia: A toxic condition of pregnancy with high blood pressure that increases, headaches, albuminuria and swelling of the lower extremities

premenopausal: Before the cessation of menses

progestational agent: Any one of several chemical substances that have the effect of progesterone. They are usually synthetic, and are used in birth control pills." Wallace Simons, R.Ph, Women's International Pharmacy.

progesterone: A natural steroid hormone found in the corpus luteum and placenta. It is responsible for changes in uterine endometrium in the second half of the menstrual cycle preparatory for implantation of the blastocyst, development of maternal placenta after implantation and development of mammary glands.

Progestins: (Synthetic) Term used to cover a large group of synthetic drugs that have a progesterone-like effect on the uterus. Used in medications like oral contraceptives. Some are synthetically derived from the male hormone, testosterone, or chemically modified from natural progesterone. Synthetic progestins can inhibit ovulation, thus suppressing the body's output of its own hormone, progesterone

Progestogens: Any natural or synthetic hormonal substance that produces effects similar to those due to progesterone

protocol: A plan to follow consisting of a series of steps; a regimen. A clinical nutrition protocol includes a list of products along with instructions for taking them over a length of time, usually 3 months

protomorphogen (PMG): The biological template for organs, made of complexes of nucleoprotein molecules, a phosphorus backbone, and a mineral substrate with as many as 60 to 90 trace minerals

resorption: The process by which a substance is dissolved or eliminated

tetany: Muscle spasms often related to parathyroid deficiency, emotional excitement or infectious fevers

transdermal: Through the skin

valence: A measure of the combining power or relative capacity of an atom to interact with a biological substrate

⟐ *Appendix*

Sources

Standard Process
1200 West Royal Lee Drive
Palmyra, Wisconsin 53156
1-800-848-5061
Fax: 414-495-2512
www.standardprocess.com

For referral to a practitioner:

Call 1-800-558-8740, or
e-mail: info@standardprocess.com

For Dr. Versendaal's audio or video library:

Cottage Video
P. O. Box 706
Bonners Ferry, Idaho 83805
208-267-3555
e-mail: www.cotvideo@dmi.net

For Dr. Versendaal's clinical nutrition reference manuals and his schedule of professional trainings:

C.R.A. and Nutrition Research Foundation
P. O. Box 914
Jenison, Michigan 49429-0914
616-669-5534
Dhoezee@i2k.com
e-mail: crahealth.org

For Dr. Dobbins' videotape library:
DPG Video
5960 S. Land Park Drive #143
Sacramento, California 95822

The Lectures of Dr. Royal Lee
published by Selene River Press 1-800-321-9807

To subscribe to Bruce West's *Health Alert:*
Health Alert
5 Harris Court, N6
Monterey, California 93940
408-372-2103

For a signed quality paperback of Jensen & Anderson's *Empty Harvest:*
Standard Process West
P. O. Box 270547
Fort Collins, Colorado 80527-0547
1-800-321-9807

Price-Pottenger Nutrition Foundation
P. O. Box 2614
La Mesa, California 91943-2614
1-800-FOODS4U
professional and lay memberships
Dr.'s referral lists for 3 states of your choice for $6.00 donation

For a catalogue of books and materials on nutrition:
International Foundation for Nutrition and Health
3963 Mission Blvd.
San Diego, California 92109
858-488-8932
fax 858-488-2566

The American Association of Naturopathic Physicians
P. O. Box 20386
Seattle, Washington 98102
206-323-7610

For Natural Progesterone Supplements:

The Women's International Pharmacy
5708 Monona Drive
Madison, Wisconsin 53716-3152

Osteoporosis and Related Bone Diseases
National Resource Center
1150 17th Street N.W. #500
Washington, D.C. 20036-4603
Funded by the National Institutes of Health

Two companies supply computerized programs to process symptom survey forms:

Nutritec Software
DPG Video
5960 S. Land Park Drive #143
Sacramento, California 95822

Symptom Survey Scheduler
Nutricom Software
54 Mott Avenue
Roslyn, New York 11576
516-625-8245
e-mail: nutricom@optonline.net

For published research on nutrition:

The American Society for Clinical Nutrition
www.faseb.org/ascn

The American Journal of Clinical Nutrition
www.faseb.org/ajcn

To find out about pollution in your area:

Enter your zipcode at
http://www.scorecard.org/community/index.
This is a service provide by the Environmental Defense Fund.

For more information on hormone disruptors:

www.epa.gov/endocrine
Also see
www.wwfcanada.org/hormone-disruptors/index.html

National Women's Health Network
51410 10th Street N.W. #400
Washington, D.C. 20004

Men's Health Consulting
Will Courtnay, Ph.D., L.C.S.W.
2811 College Avenue, Suite 1
Berkeley, California 94705-2167
1-800-WELL MEN
www.menshealth.org

provides education to health professionals, worksites and colleges addressing behaviors and beliefs that damage men's health, including beliefs about manhood.

To add your voice and support for the right to know personal health care information, contact:

Citizens for Health, Defending Your Right to Choose
P. O. Box 2260
Boulder, Colorado 80306
800-357-2211
www.citzens.org

For Standard Process products from non-U.S. locations:

Justin Toal
Standard Process of Northern California
1000 Atlantic Blvd. Suite 109
Alameda, California 94501
510-865-4322
info@spnatural.com

Bibliography

American Council on Collaborative Medicine, Vol. IV, Issue 5, May 1998.

Atkins, Robert C., M.D. *Dr. Atkins' New Diet Revolution*, Avon Health, New York, New York, 1997.

Appleton, Nancy. *Healthy Bones, What You Should Know about Osteoporosis*, Avery, Garden City Park, New York, 1991.

Balch, James, M.D., and Phyllis A. Balch, C.N.C. *Prescription for Nutritional Healing*, Second Edition, Avery, Garden City, New Jersey, 1997.

Barilla, Jean, M.S. "Rx for Health Care" in *The Physicians Newsletter, Health through Nutrition*, Jones Medical Industries, Inc., St. Louis, Missouri, Vol. 2, No. 1, April 1997.

Baurac, Deborah. "Joint Exchange" in *Modern Maturity*, September-October 1997.

Bendavid, E. J., J. Shan, and E. Barrett-Conner. "Factors Associated with Bone Mineral Density in Middle-Aged Men." *Journal of Bone Mineral Research*, 11, No. 8, August 1996.

Biondo, Brenda. "Are common chemicals scrambling your hormones?" in *U.S.A. Weekend*, Feb. 13–15, 1998.

Black, Dean. "Artful Science: Documenting the Chiropractic Experience," Parker College, Occasional Paper, 1996, 1, as quoted in Clecak, Ph.D., "Giving Patients 'Reasonable Counsel': The Case of Contact Reflex Analysis."

Bodmer, Kerry. *Osteoporosis and the Calcium Controversy*. Soundview Publications, Inc., Atlanta, Georgia, 1996.

_____. *Got Milk? Get Heart Disease*. Soundview Publications, Inc., Atlanta, Georgia, 1996.

_____. "Don't Let New Fosamex Study Fool You" in *Women's Health Letter*, Vol. VII, No. 4, April 1998.

_____. "Editronate and Osteoporosis" in *Women's Health Letter*, Vol. VII, No. 5, May 1998.

_____. "Healthy Body, Healthy Bones" in *Women's Health Letter*, Vol. VI, No. 7, July 1998.

_____. "Health Secrets for Women Only" in *Women's Health News*, supplement, October 1998.

_____. "Update on Calcium Channel Blockers" in *Women's Health Letter*, Vol. VII, No. 5, May 1998.

_____. with Nan Kathryn Fuchs. *Stop Breast Cancer Before It Happens*. Soundview Publications, Inc., Atlanta, Georgia, 1997.

Bortz, Sharon, R.D. "Boning Up on Calcium" in *Redwood Health Club Newsletter*, September 1997.

_____. "Calcium, Part 3" in *Redwood Health Club Newsletter*, November 1997.

Brown, Susan E., Ph.D. *Better Bones, Better Body*. Keats Publishing Company, New Canaan, Conneticut, 1996.

Carper, Jean. "Calcium: Not for women only" in *U.S.A. Weekend*, March 27–29, 1997.

"Calcium, Beneficial to Bones and More" in *Healthy Cell News*, Spring/Summer 1996.

Clecak, Peter, Ph.D, Ron Carsten, D.V.M., M.S., Paul Jasoviak, D.C., Mary Jane Mack, R.N., Steve Nelson, Pharm.D., Ph.D., Michael Robertson, M.D., J. Rodney Shelley, D.C., Donald Warren, D.D.S., F.A.H.N.P., "Alternative Healing Modes, A Look at Contact Reflex Analysis" in *Alternative Medicine Journal*, July/August 1994.

Colgan, Dr. Michael. *Hormonal Health, Nutritional and Hormonal Strategies for Emotional Well-being and Intellectual Longevity*, Apple Publishing, Vancouver, British Columbia, Canada, 1996.

Courtney, John and Royal Lee. *Conversations in Nutrition*, unpublished notes from question and answer sessions with health professionals.

D'Adamo, Peter. *Eat Right For Your Type*, Riverhead/Putnam, New York, 1996.

DeCava, Judith A., M.S., L.N.C. *The Real Truth about Vitamins and Antioxidants*, Brentwood Academic Press, Columbus, Georgia, 1996.

Deets, Horace B. "A.A.R.P.'s Realignment" in AARP Perspectives, *Modern Maturity*, November–December 1997.

Douglass, William Campbell, M.D. "Say Goodbye to Illness" in *Health Breakthroughs*, Fall 1997.

_____. "Astonishing New Cure Reverses Osteoporosis" in *Health Breakthroughs*, Winter 1997.

_____. "Steps Toward Beating Osteoporosis" in *Second Opinion*, November 1995.

Dover, Clare. *Osteoporosis*, Ward Lock in conjunction with the National Osteoporosis Society, London, England, 1994.

Dufty, William. *Sugar Blues*, Warner Books, New York, 1975.

Eades, Michael R., M.D., and Mary Dan Eades, M.D. *Protein Power*, Bantam, New York, 1998.

Flaherty, Megan, "Healthy Planet, Hospitals learn to clean up their act" in *NurseWeek*, Vol. 12, No. 2, p. 1, Jan. 25, 1999.

Frost, Mary, M.A. *Going Back to the Basics of Human Health, Avoiding the Fads, the Trends and the Bold-Faced Lies*, self-published, February 1997.

Fuchs, Nan Kathryn, Ph.D. "The Nutrition Detective" in *Women's Health Letter*, Vol. VII, No. 4, April 1998.

Gaby, Alan, M.D. *Preventing and Reversing Osteoporosis, Every Woman's Essential Guide*, Prima Publishing, Rocklin, California, 1994.

Gittleman, Anne Louise, M.S. *Beyond Pritikin*, Bantam Books, New York, New York, 1989, as quoted in www.barleans.com/flax.html.

Green, Jerry, J.D. "Collaborative physician-patient planning and professional liability: Opening the legal door to unconventional medicine" in *Advances in Mind-Body Medicine*, Vol. 15, No. 2, Spring 1999.

_____. "The Health Care Contract: A Model for Sharing Responsibility" from *The New Holistic Health Handbook—1985* as revised from *Somatics*, Vol. 3, No. 4., 1982.

Griggs, Barbara. *Green Pharmacy*, Healing Arts Press, Rochester, Vermont, 1997.

Harrower, Henry R., M.D. *Practical Endocrinology*, Second Edition, Lee Foundation for Nutritional Research, Milwaukee, Wisconsin, 1957.

Hellinghausen, Mary Ann, Leigh Morgan, and Valeria J. Nelson for *NurseWeek*, June 23, 1997.

Hermann, Mindy. "A Call for Calcium" in *Modern Maturity*, March-April 1998.

Higashida, George. Letter, Sun Wellness, Inc.

http://www.os2bbs.com/malka/osteopRX.htm

http://www.vvv.com./healthnews/dvitamin.html

Jackson, Donna M. *The Bone Detectives: How Forensic Anthropologists Solve Crimes and Uncover Mysteries of the Dead*, Little, 1996.

Jackson, Mildred, N.D., and Terri Teague. *The Handbook of Alternatives to Chemical Medicine*. Oakland, California, 1975.

Jensen, Bernard, and Mark Anderson. *Empty Harvest, Understanding the Link Between Our Food, Our Immunity, and Our Planet*. Avery Publishing Group, Inc., Garden City Park, New York, 1990.

Journal of the American Dietetic Association: www.columbia.net/consumer/datafile/osteo.html. March 1995.

Lanucci, Lisa. "Bone Power" in *Energy Times*, May 1997.

Lee, John, M.D. "Osteoporosis Reversal The Role of Progesterone" in *The International Clinical Nutrition Review*, Vol. 10, No. 3, July 1990.

_____. *Natural Progesterone, The Multiple Roles of a Remarkable Hormone*, BLL Publishing, Sebastopol, California, 1993.

_____. with Virginia Hopkins. *What Your Doctor May Not Tell You about Menopause, The Breakthrough Book on Natural Progesterone*. Warner, New York, 1996.

Lee, Royal, D.D.S. *The Principles of Cell Auto-Regulation*, 1947.

_____. *Therapeutic Food Manual*. Publication date unknown.

_____. "Food Integrity" in *Conversations in Nutrition*, April 1955.

LeRoy, Bob, R.D. "Major Study Results Challenge Claims for Dairy" in *Vegetarian Voice*, Autumn 1997.

Levin, Alan S., M.S. M.D., J.D. Author's Interview, May 1998.

Martin, Claire. "A Positive Impact," *Outside*, December 1997.

Miller, Glenn, M.D. "What are some benefits from exposure to sunlight?" *Ukiah Daily Journal*.

Murray, Michael, N.D. "The *true* arthritis cure" in *The Arthritis Counselor*, Special Edition, 1997.

National Osteoporosis Foundation. "Men with Osteoporosis, in their own words." National Osteoporosis Foundation, Washington, D.C., 1997.

Natural vs. Synthetic (Is Natural Better?) in *The Nu Pro Therapist*, MPI NUPRO, Volume II Number II.

NIH Consensus Statement, National Institutes of Health, Office of the Director, Volume 12, Number 4, June 6-8, 1994.

Northrup, Christiane, M.D. *Women's Bodies, Women's Wisdom, Creating Physical and Emotional Health and Healing*, Bantam, March, New York, 1998.

Optimal Calcium Intake, National Institutes of Health Continuing Medical Education Consensus Statement, Volume 12 Number 4, June 6-8 1994.

Osteoporosis and Related Bone Diseases National Resource Center, National Osteoporosis Foundation, National Institutes of Health, Washington, D.C., June 1996 and July 1997.

Osteoporosis and You, Colorado Department of Health, Osteo-
    porosis Prevention Project, PPD-IP-A5, Denver, Colorado,
    Vol. 1, No. 3.

Paterson, Jim. "Is there 'male menopause'?" in *USA Weekend*,
    Jan. 2–4, 1998.

Percival, Mark. "Bone Health and Osteoporosis" *Clinical Nutri-
    tion Insights*, Vol. 5, No. 4, 1998.

Price-Pottenger Foundation Newsletter from *Acupuncture and
    Electro-Therapeutics* Res Int J, 20: 1995.

Price, Westin. *Nutrition and Physical Degeneration*, Price-Pottenger
    Nutritional Foundation, La Mesa, California, 1939.

Prior, J.C. "Progesterone as a Bone-Trophic Hormone" in
    Endocrine Reviews, Vol. 11, No. 2, May 1990.

Quillman, Susan M., R.N., M.N. *Nutrition and Diet Therapy*,
    Second Edition, Springhouse Notes, Springhouse, Pennsyl-
    vania. 1994.

Reid, I. R., and others. "Testosterone Therapy in Glucocorti-
    coid-Treated Men." *Archives of Internal Medicine*, 156, No.
    11, June 1996.

Robbins, John. *Reclaiming Our Health, Exploding the Medical
    Myth and Embracing the Source of True Healing*, H. J. Kramer,
    Tiburon, California, 1996.

Rosenfeld, Isadore, M.D. *Dr. Rosenfeld's Guide to Alternative
    Medicine*, Random House, New York, 1996.

Schmidt, D. Raymond. "A Treatment for Leprosy" in *Health Jour-
    nal*, Price-Pottenger Nutrition Foundation, Vol. 21, No. 3.

Shaner, Hollie, M.S.A., R.N. Interview, *NurseWeek*, April 19,
    1999.

Sheehy, Gail. *New Passages, Mapping Your Life Across Time*,
    Random House, New York, 1995.

Shefi, Ron. "Contact Reflex Analysis" in *C.R.A. Collector's Edition*.

Simons, Wallace, R.Ph. "A Pharmacist Explores Some Differ-
    ences Between Natural Progesterone and Synthetic Prog-
    estins" in *Women's Health Connections*, Issue IIb, 1997.

Smatt, Dr. Michael. "Gloria Steinem" in *Today's Chiropractic*, March/April 1996.

"Sulfur an Ancient Nutrient Needed Now, More Than Ever Before" in *American Council on Collaborative Medicine*, Volume IV, Issue 3, March 1998.

Supplee, G., Ansbacher, S., Bender, R., and Flinigan, G. *Journal of Biological Chemistry*, 141, 1:95-107, May 1936.

Taber's Cyclopedic Medical Dictionary, Eighth Edition, F. A. David Company, Philadelphia, 1960.

The Complete Book of Natural and Medicinal Cures, How to Choose the Most Potent Healing Agents for over 300 Conditions and Diseases, eds., *Prevention* Magazine health books, Rodale Press, Emmaus, Pennsylvania, 1994.

The New Medicine Show, Consumers Union's new practical guide to some everyday health products by the editors of Consumer Reports Books, Mount Vernon, New York, 1989.

The Whole Truth About Vitamins, audiotape, Health America, 1997.

Therapeutic Food Manual, an unpublished compilation of nutritional information gathered from health care practitioners.

Theodosakis, Jason, M.D., M.S., M.P.H., Brenda Adderly, M.H.A., and Barry Fox, Ph.D. *The Arthritis Cure*, St. Martin's Press, New York, 1997.

Ulan, Fred, D.C., C.C.N. "Preventing Recurring Subluxations with CRA" in *The American Chiropractor*, September-October 1998.

Versendaal, D.A., and Dawn Versendaal Hoeze. *CRA and Designed Clinical Nutrition*, Hoeze Marketing, 1993.

Versendaal, D.A., D.C. "C.R.A. Technology and Osteoporosis, The 'Brittle Bone' Syndrome," Contact Reflex Analysis Seminar Papers, Summer 1998.

Wardlaw, Gordon M. "Putting Body Weight and Osteoporosis into Perspective," *American Journal of Clinical Nutrition*, March 1996; 63 (suppl. 433-6S.)

West, Bruce. *Health Alert*, Vol. 14, Issue 7, July 1997.

_____. Vol. 14, Issue 9, September, 1997.

_____. Vol. 15, Issue 2, February 1998.

_____. Vol. 15, Issue 5, May 1998.

_____. Vol. 15, Issue 7, July 1998.

_____. Vol. 15, Issue 9, August 1998.

Wyeth-Ayerst Laboratories advertisement, *USA Weekend* Magazine, September 26-28, 1997.

Whitaker, Julian, M.D. "Health Breakthroughs", *Second Opinion*, Atlanta, Georgia, Spring 1998.

www.cspinet.org/new/olesnatl.htm

www.xs4all.nl/hempy/hemp.htm

www.pathfinder.com/time/magazine/archive/1994/940905/94090

Yiamouyiannis, John, Ph.D. "Lifesavers Guide to Fluoridation, Risks/Benefits Evaluated", a report published by the Safe Water Foundation, Delaware, Ohio, 1988.

Yost, Hunter, M.D. *Molecules for the Mind*, www.azstarnet.com/healthbeat/mole.htm.

❧ About the Author

PAMELA LEVIN, R.N., is an award-winning author. In writing this book as a nutritional journalist, she draws on over 30 years' experience in the health field. She compiled *Perfect Bones* out of gratitude after recovering her own bone health using the methods described in these pages.

She is a graduate of the University of Illinois College of Nursing, Chicago, has over 70 hours of postgraduate education in advanced clinical nutrition, and is a practitioner of Contact Reflex Analysis.™

She studied Transactional Analysis with its founder, Eric Berne, and became the first nurse to be awarded Clinical, then Teaching Membership in its international organization. She has taught and trained health professionals in 51 U.S. cities and in 6 foreign countries on 4 continents.

Her other writings, now in ten languages, include numerous published articles and four books which have sold over 100,000 copies worldwide. Her books *Becoming the Way We Are* and *Cycles of Power* received the Eric Berne Memorial Scientific Award, and are the foundation for Jean Illsley Clarke's parent education system, *Self-Esteem, a Family Affair* and *Growing Up Again*, as well as John Bradshaw's book and PBS series, *Homecoming*.

She has been in private practice since 1970. She is the mother of 2 grown children.

≈ Index

Other Titles Available from The Nourishing Company

Cycles of Power, A User's Guide to the Seven Seasons of Life. Shows how we can successfully navigate the cyclic transitions of life. Includes exercises.

Les Cycles de l'identite. French language version of *Cycles of Power* published by InterEditions, Paris.

Becoming the Way We Are, A Transactional Guide to Personal Development. A Clear and encouraging summary of the growing stages of life begun in childhood and repeated in the cycle of adult life. Outlines how to make peace with common developmental issues.

How to Develop Your Personal Powers, A Workbook for Your Life's Time. A personal workbook for identifying the key issues for each of your developmental stages and what to do to grow beyond them.

The Fuzzy Frequency, a delightful coloring book about affection and positive strokes for children of all ages. Illustrations by Sunny Mehler.

For a complete listing of books, materials, products and services, send your name and address to The Nourishing Company, P.O. Box 1429, Ukiah, California 95482

To order additional copies of this book, send your name, shipping address, city, state, zip and phone number along with check or money order for $39.95 per copy plus $4.00 shipping per copy (add $3.00 tax per copy if shipped to California address or enclose resale number)

To: The Nourishing Company
P.O. Box 1429
Ukiah, California 95482

Quantity discount information available on request.

We welcome your comments.